Working with Families
of Psychiatric Inpatients

Working with Families
of Psychiatric Inpatients

A *Guide for Clinicians*

ALISON M. HERU, M.D.
Associate Professor (Clinical)
and
LAURA M. DRURY, M.S.W., L.I.C.S.W.
Senior Clinical Teaching Associate

Department of Psychiatry and Human Behavior
Brown University Medical School
Providence, Rhode Island

The Johns Hopkins University Press
Baltimore

© 2007 The Johns Hopkins University Press
All rights reserved. Published 2007
Printed in the United States of America on acid-free paper

2   4   6   8   9   7   5   3   1

The Johns Hopkins University Press
2715 North Charles Street
Baltimore, Maryland 21218-4363
www.press.jhu.edu

Library of Congress Cataloging-in-Publication Data
Heru, Alison M., 1953–
Working with families of psychiatric inpatients : a guide for
clinicians / Alison M. Heru and Laura M. Drury.
p. ; cm.
Includes bibliographical references and index.
ISBN-13: 978-0-8018-8576-1 (hardcover : alk. paper)
ISBN-10: 0-8018-8576-0 (hardcover : alk. paper)
ISBN-13: 978-0-8018-8577-8 (pbk. : alk. paper)
ISBN-10: 0-8018-8577-9 (pbk. : alk. paper)
1. Psychiatric hospital care. 2. Family—Mental health. I. Drury,
Laura M., 1948–   II. Title.
[DNLM: 1. Mental Disorders—therapy. 2. Family Relations.
3. Hospitalization. 4. Internship and Residency. 5. Professional-
Family Relations. WM 140 H576w 2007]
RC439.W6744 2007
362.2'1—dc22
2006026088

A catalog record for this book is available from the British Library.

Contents

Preface

The primary goal of this book is to provide guidance to clinicians who are working with psychiatric inpatients and their families. The book offers step-by-step instruction for successfully working with families. It can be useful to psychiatric residents and trainees in other disciplines who want to learn how to provide good family-oriented care to mentally ill patients and their families.

Another reason for writing this book is the expectation that residents in all specialties will be competent in working with families. This expectation is clearly laid out in the core competencies of the Accreditation Council for General Medical Education. Residents will be assessed on their knowledge, attitudes, and skills in working with families. The Psychiatric Residency Review Committee has amplified these criteria for psychiatry, and the Committee on the Family of the Group for the Advancement of Psychiatry has fleshed out these criteria to make implementation easier. The criteria are presented in Chapter 1.

Beyond meeting competency expectations, however, the stronger rationale for working with families comes from the broad and deep research on families that exists throughout the medical literature. The research data clearly demonstrate why family interventions are important for patient care. Research on families and evidence-based family treatments that are relevant to inpatient care is described in Chapters 3 and 4. The biopsychosocial model is discussed in Chapter 2, as it is considered an exemplary model for integrating family factors into the assessment and treatment of patients.

Chapters 5, 6, and 7 outline the attitudes and skills necessary for the clinician to be able to assess and treat families successfully. Case material, including teaching points, is used to illustrate these skills. The cases are loosely based on families that we have worked with in an inpatient setting.

While the names and details have been changed, of course, the lessons learned remain authentic.

The chapters in Part 4, "Challenges in Working with Families," outline the barriers that clinicians may encounter with families. Chapter 8 contains case examples that illustrate concerns residents have brought to us during their training. Families also bring fears and anxieties to a family meeting, and Chapter 9 and its case example help attune the reader to the concerns of the family. Understanding the family's perspective enhances the clinician's capacity for empathy with the family, allowing him or her to intervene more effectively.

Part 5 provides a wider view of the importance of families in psychiatric care. In Chapter 10, Dr. Patricia Recupero, the vice president of the American Academy of Psychiatry and the Law and the president and CEO of Butler Hospital, in Providence, Rhode Island, offers a legal perspective on the importance of involving families in patient care. Using legal case material, she discusses risk-management strategies as part of a model of patient care that is family oriented. The final chapter places the concerns of the family within a community perspective and reviews how mental health services, if adequately funded, can continue family-oriented care beyond hospitalization.

Family skills should be part of the repertoire of every clinician. We do not suggest that every resident become a family therapist, but all residents should develop skills that will allow them to easily integrate the family into patient care. This book offers guidance on how to manage family situations that are commonly encountered on the inpatient unit and demonstrates why clinicians should welcome family involvement in patient care. When the skills of working with families are incorporated into a clinician's repertoire, they will counterbalance the recent trend of psychiatrists to become psychopharmacologists. As one former chief resident stated in a letter to the *Psychiatric Times*, "Why would a fully trained psychiatrist want to diminish 4 years of biopsychosocial training by emphasizing only the training in medications? Psychopharmacologists are inherently consultants, focusing on one small piece of the biopsychosocial puzzle—and interestingly, perhaps the smallest piece. For as any psychiatric resident can attest, learning the meds is the easiest piece. The richness, complexity, artistry and joy of our specialty come from understanding and optimizing the interaction between our patients and ourselves" (Heacock 2004, p. 13). To this, we would add that interactions with the patients' families are another arena in which psychiatrists can experience the richness and artistry of our profession and optimize patient care.

We gratefully acknowledge the contributions to Chapter 1 of the GAP Committee on the Family members (Ellen Berman, Alison Heru, John Rolland, Fred Gottleib, Henry Grunebaum, Beatrice Wood, and Heidi Bruty). The chapter is adapted from an article published in *Academic Psychiatry* in 2005. We thank our supervisors, Drs. Nathan Epstein and Duane Bishop, for guidance throughout our training years. We thank Jody Eyre, a marital and family therapy intern from the University of Rhode Island, who piloted genogram groups at Butler Hospital. Finally, we thank the families of our patients for making our work easier and for the trust they place in us.

This book is dedicated to our own families, in recognition of their support and encouragement.

Abbreviations

ACGME	Accreditation Council for General Medical Education
APA	American Psychiatric Association
BPS	biopsychosocial (model)
EE	expressed emotion
EOI	emotional overinvolvement
FFEP	Family-to-Family Education Program
GAP	Group for the Advancement of Psychiatry
GARF	Global Assessment of Relational Functioning
MIRECC	Mental Illness Research, Education and Clinical Center
MMFF	McMaster Model of Family Functioning
NAMI	National Alliance for the Mentally Ill
RRC	Residency Review Committee
SAFE	Support and Family Education (Program)

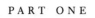

PART ONE

Key Concepts

CHAPTER ONE

What It Takes to Work
with Patients' Families

This chapter outlines the knowledge, skills, and attitudes necessary for a clinician to provide a family-oriented approach to inpatient psychiatric care. The chapter illustrates how residents can meet the expected level of competence in these skills and discusses the assessment of residents' progress in competency.

In current practice on an inpatient psychiatric unit, brief assessment of patients and quick resolution of acute symptoms is the standard of care. The shortening of hospital stays and the lack of funding for community psychiatry have resulted in families' bearing the brunt of caring for a patient after discharge from the hospital. Family members are unsure of how to proceed. When given the opportunity, they often ask the psychiatrist basic questions such as, "Should we be quiet around her when she comes home? Does she need to rest? Can she go back to work? What should I do if she cries or gets upset? What do I do if she refuses to get out of bed or if she won't take her medication? Should she be able to take her medication on her own? Do I need to watch for anything? Will she try to kill herself again? What is the risk that this illness is inherited and other family members may become ill?" Currently, families receive little information about what to expect and how best to care for a relative after discharge. Psychiatric residents often state that they do not know how to help family members and are afraid of giving the wrong advice.

Unfortunately, on the inpatient unit, clinicians often see patients' families as an intrusion: family members often want to speak to the resident or the nurse at visiting times, and their need for time and attention may seem insatiable. Often it is the least-experienced staff member, such as the medical student or resident, who has to "deal with the family." Without adequate training, the resident may tend to dodge family members, rather than engage them in a productive way.

THE SIX CORE COMPETENCIES

Medical educators have recognized that physicians need to have more humanistic skills to meet the needs of patients and their families in the current managed care environment. The Accreditation Council for General Medical Education (ACGME) developed a set of six core competencies that apply to all medical specialities; the council will require residency programs to show that residents meet these competencies before graduation (ACGME 2004). The six core areas in which competency must be demonstrated are patient care, medical knowledge, interpersonal and communication skills, systems-based practice, professionalism, and practice-based learning and improvement. Families are involved in five of the six core competencies. For example, in demonstrating interpersonal and communication skills, residents are asked to show their ability to educate patients, their families, and other professionals about medical, psychosocial, and behavioral issues. Residents are expected to develop a working alliance with patients and their families and to ensure that the patient and/or family have understood the communication. For family psychiatrists who use systems theory in their work with families (Bertalanffy 1968), the competency referred to as systems-based practice holds great potential for teaching about family systems.

The Residency Review Committee for psychiatry specified the core competencies as they apply to psychiatry (a summary of them is given in Table 1.1). In order to meet these core competencies, psychiatric residents need to be able to assess the patient's position within the family and the larger social system, to formulate a treatment plan that includes these psychosocial elements, and to support the family system and educate family members. The inpatient unit provides an excellent opportunity for the resi-

TABLE 1.1
Core Competencies Specific to Family and Systems Issues in Psychiatry

Patient Care: Based on a relevant psychiatric assessment, physicians shall demonstrate the following abilities:

1. to develop and document an appropriate DSM-IV multiaxial differential diagnosis; an integrative case formulation that includes neurobiological, phenomenological, psychological, and sociocultural issues involved in diagnosis and management; a comprehensive treatment plan addressing biological, psychological, and sociocultural domains.
2. to conduct a range of individual, group, and family therapies using standard accepted models and to integrate these psychotherapies in multimodal treatment, including biological and sociocultural interventions.

Medical Knowledge: Knowledge of major disorders, including considerations relating to age, gender, race, and ethnicity, based on the literature and standards of practice. This knowledge shall include:

1. the etiology of the disorder, including medical, genetic, and sociocultural factors.
2. the experience, meaning, and explanation of the illness for the patient and family, including the influence of cultural factors and culture-bound syndromes.

Interpersonal and Communication Skills: Physicians shall demonstrate the following abilities: to educate patients, their families, and professionals about medical, psychosocial, and behavioral issues. This shall include discussing the consultation findings with the patient and family. Physicians shall demonstrate the ability to communicate effectively with patients and their families by:

1. gearing all communication to the educational and intellectual levels of patients and their families.
2. demonstrating sociocultural sensitivity to patients and their families.
3. providing explanations of psychiatric and neurological disorders and treatment that are jargon free and geared to the educational/intellectual levels of patients and their families.
4. providing preventive education that is understandable and practical.
5. developing and enhancing rapport and a working alliance with patients and their families.
6. ensuring that the patient and/or family have understood the communication.

In addition, physicians shall demonstrate the ability to obtain, interpret, and evaluate consultations from other medical specialties.

Professionalism: Physicians shall demonstrate respect for patients, their families, and colleagues as persons, including their ages, cultures, disabilities, ethnicities, genders, socioeconomic backgrounds, religious beliefs, political leanings, and sexual orientations.

Systems-Based Practice: Physicians should have a working knowledge of the diverse systems involved in treating patients of all ages and should understand how to use the systems as part of a comprehensive system of care in general and as part of a comprehensive, individualized treatment plan.

Source: Group for the Advancement of Psychiatry, Committee on the Family 2006.

dent to attain these competencies while being closely supervised. Teaching family skills early in the resident's professional career ensures that the resident will integrate these skills into his or her work as a matter of routine.

The Committee on the Family of the Group for the Advancement of Psychiatry (GAP), a psychiatric think tank, has chosen the teaching of family skills in psychiatric residency programs as its current educational priority. The GAP Committee on the Family developed a set of family skills for residents based on the RRC requirements. The GAP criteria provide clear and measurable expectations for residents and their supervisors in their work with patients and families (Table 1.2). It is hoped that, with a clear set of expectations for the teaching of family skills, residency programs will find it relatively easy to incorporate the teaching and assessment of these skills into their curricula.

A major shift in thinking is occurring among family psychiatrists. The new emphasis is on teaching residents how to interact effectively with patients' families in any treatment setting, rather than concentrating on teaching family therapy. For example, contact with the family in the emergency room establishes a hospital experience that is family-oriented, is respectful of the family, and encourages a good working relationship among the patient, the family, and the treatment team. Several of the core competency requirements are needed in the emergency room encounter: the ability to develop a therapeutic alliance with the family (interpersonal and communication skills), showing respect for culturally diverse patients and families (professionalism), and educating the patient and family concerning the inpatient system of care (systems-based practice). Psychiatric residency programs can incorporate the attainment of these competencies into the expectations of the emergency psychiatry rotation.

Attainment of these core competencies is illustrated in the following typical emergency room encounter. A resident interviews the patient and the family together. After introductions, the resident explains the procedure: "I will ask questions about why you are here, give you an assessment of the problem, and then discuss treatment options." If sensitive issues emerge, the resident can defer discussion of these issues until there is an opportunity for privacy or, if the material is judged to be essential to the presenting complaint, the resident can ask the family to step out. After discussion of the sensitive material, the family would be invited back into the room. If

TABLE 1.2

Knowledge: The resident is expected to demonstrate knowledge of family factors as they relate to psychiatric and nonpsychiatric disorders, based on scientific literature and standards of practice. The resident is expected to demonstrate knowledge of the following:

1. basic concepts of systems applicable to families, multidisciplinary teams in clinical settings, and medical/governmental organizations affecting the patient and doctor.
2. couple and family development over the life cycle and the importance of multigenerational patterns.
3. principles of adaptive and maladaptive relational functioning in family life: family organization, communication, problem solving, and emotional regulation.
4. family strengths, resilience, and vulnerability.
5. how age, gender, class, culture, and spirituality affect family life.
6. the variety of family forms (single parent, stepfamily, same-sex parents, etc.).
7. how the family affects and is affected by psychiatric and nonpsychiatric disorders. This includes specific information regarding the impact of parental psychiatric illness on children.
8. special issues in family life, including loss, divorce and remarriage, immigration, illness, secrets, affairs, violence, alcohol and substance abuse, sexuality (including gay, lesbian, bisexual, and transsexual issues).
9. relationship of families to larger systems (e.g., schools, work, health care systems, governmental agencies).

Attitudes: The attitudes held and demonstrated by the competent resident are empathy, curiosity, and respect for all family members. The resident must accept differences in perspectives on the problem and solution and understand that, in families, there is no ultimate "truth." This is demonstrated by:

1. allowing each family member to describe the presenting problem.
2. identifying and acknowledging strengths and prior attempts at problem solving.
3. acknowledging realistic limitations while maintaining an attitude of hopefulness.
4. showing balanced concern for each member of the family and his or her point of view.
5. working collaboratively with families and seeing them as allies.

Skills: The resident should demonstrate reasonable ability to conduct a family interview and to complete an assessment and formulation that includes family factors. Operational skills include:

1. Identify family members and other relevant persons in larger systems who are involved with the patient's current functioning. In adult residency programs, this might include parents, spouses, partners, adults or children, extended family, and staff in health care and other systems.
2. Meet with patient's significant family members and be able to deal with reluctance on the part of patient or family to meet.
3. Foster a therapeutic alliance with all family members by instilling feelings of trust, openness, and rapport.

(*continued*)

4. In an assessment interview, the resident should:
   a. elicit each family member's perspective of the presenting problem.
   b. obtain a family history, including strengths, stressors, and repeating inter-generational patterns of behavior or illness. The ability to construct a genogram and a time line is helpful in this process.
   c. elicit the family's culture, class, etc., and describe how these affect their response to the patient and his or her illness and treatment.
   d. identify and asses the emotional climate, family organization, and inter-actional problem solving as described by the GARF. Include the GARF score in assessment.
   e. be aware of personal feelings in relation to family members and be able to tolerate and work effectively in the presence of intense affects, especially when directed at the resident.
   f. elicit strengths, competencies, and resources of couples and families so that they become useful and effective allies in treatment.
5. Following the interview, the resident should be able to:
   a. integrate the impact of current relational functioning into the case formulation.
   b. present the case formulation and, if appropriate, psychoeducation to the family in a frame that is respectful, culturally acceptable, and comprehensible.
   c. involve the family members in collaborative treatment planning. Support the family in resolving differences of opinions with family members regarding treatment.
   d. make recommendations for interventions which may include other members of the system, such as the treatment of depression in the spouse.

For each of the core competencies, the level of expertise is as follows:
1. In patient care, the resident must demonstrate the ability to perform and document an adequate sociocultural and family history and to formulate a treatment plan that includes sociocultural aspects.
2. In medical knowledge, the resident must demonstrate knowledge of the experience, meaning, and explanation of the illness for the patient and the family. In addition, the resident should understand the family factors associated with specific illnesses, such as genetic implications, caregiver burden associated with chronic illness, and the normal developmental stages of the family.
3. In interpersonal and communication skills, the resident must demonstrate the ability to listen to and understand family members, communicate effectively about the treatment plan with the patient and family, and provide patient/family education. These communications should be jargon free and geared to their educational/intellectual level and be respectful of the family's cultural, ethnic, and economic background and identity and their impact on the experience, meaning, and evaluation of the illness. Residents must demonstrate the ability to develop a working alliance with the patients and their families.

(*continued*)

TABLE 1.2
GAP Proposal for Specific Competencies in Family Systems (continued)

4. In practice-based learning and improvement, the resident must demonstrate the ability to assess the generalizability or applicability of research findings to specific patients and the families.
5. In professionalism, the resident must demonstrate respect for culturally diverse patients and their families and be able to differentiate their own experiences from those of the family.
6. In systems-based practice, the resident should be able to educate patients and their families concerning systems of care.

Source: Group for the Advancement of Psychiatry, Committee on the Family 2006, pp. 70–71.

the patient needs to be admitted against his or her will, the resident explains the process to the patient and family. If the patient is violent or dangerous, then, of course, safety concerns override all other concerns. After the admission is arranged, the resident asks the patient to sign a release of information, to allow further family contact by the psychiatrist. If the patient is unable or refuses to sign a release of information, the resident explains to the family that the inpatient team will continue to encourage the patient to sign the release. The resident educates the patient and family about what to expect during an inpatient stay. "In this hospital, inpatient stays are short, for stabilization and diagnostic assessment, usually 5–7 days. On discharge, the patient may continue to have symptoms but is considered well enough to continue treatment in a day program or an outpatient program."

This initial interview with the family is the best time to ascertain if specific issues (for example, dietary restrictions, religious needs, specific visiting arrangements) need to be taken into account to make treatment proceed smoothly. If possible, the family accompanies the patient to the psychiatric inpatient unit and receives contact telephone numbers and information about visiting times. The admitting nurse encourages the family to call later to check on their relative. Families do not benefit from psychoeducational material at the time of admission because they are usually too distressed to listen. Family members say they want a compassionate and caring attitude at the time of admission (N. Sahlin, executive director, National Alliance for the Mentally Ill, Rhode Island, personal communication, 2001).

Educators in family medicine residency programs have taught residents basic family skills for many years (Doherty 1995). In family medicine, five graded skill levels for residents are recognized:

LEVEL 1: minimal emphasis on the family

LEVEL 2: open to engaging families and providing ongoing medical information and advice

LEVEL 3: empathic listening, attentive to feelings, normalizing, identifying dysfunction, and supporting coping skills

LEVEL 4: systematic assessment and planned intervention, skill in managing family interactions and recognizing dysfunctional patterns

LEVEL 5: family therapy

It is important to see in every clinical setting the opportunity for interacting with families. For basic family skills, all teaching faculty members should be able to show and to teach up to level 3. Simple interactions with the family, such as an exchange of information, showing respect, and a willingness to develop an alliance, are skills that all physician teachers should possess. At a minimum, the resident should be expected to meet with the family, provide education, and include the family in the treatment-planning process. Supervisors with some expertise in family skills can teach level 4 skills to third- and fourth-year residents, but teaching level 5 skills requires expertise in family therapy. Community-based nonphysician adjunct faculty members can provide excellent supervision for family work with third- and fourth-year residents at levels 4 and 5.

ASSESSMENT OF RESIDENTS

The ACGME (2004) provides a toolbox of assessment methods that includes chart-stimulated recall, checklists, standardized patients, and resident portfolios. The process of assessing the resident's family skills is no different from the process for assessing ability and skill at working with individual patients. It involves evaluating the resident's ability to engage the family, understand their concerns, communicate clearly with them, and educate them as to how the illness will affect the family. The assessment process will vary depending on the resident's year of training and the goals for the rotation. For example, at level 2, a list of the number of family meetings might suffice as evidence for meeting competence. At levels 3 and 4, more extensive evaluation is necessary. As the resident's skill level increases, the evaluator will need to observe family interviews. On the inpatient unit, the assessment of family-interviewing skills is easily achieved by direct observation, like the observation of patient-interviewing skills. Outreach to the family, either by telephone or by meeting informally during visiting hours, often precedes the formal meeting. A resident's positive attitude toward families is reflected in a willingness to include the family in the patient assessment and treatment process. A "360°" global rating, which includes observations by nurses and social workers, can be used to capture the resident's achievement of this attitude. A family satisfaction questionnaire solicits the family's assessment of the resident's respect and ability to communicate and provide support and information. Checklists can also be used to document family skills; sample checklists are provided in the Appendix at the back of this volume.

Knowledge about research on families, including evidence-based treatments, family development, and systems theory, can easily be assessed by documenting attendance at seminars or completion of assigned readings. The application of knowledge can be assessed during case discussion or chart-stimulated recall. The ability to map a genogram can be considered an essential skill and provides an easy aid to patient care when placed in the patient's chart (DeMaria, Weeks, and Hof 1999; Wachtel and Wachtel 1986). As an overall goal in the assessment of patients, residents need to show that they can answer questions about family functioning, such as: What is the family's developmental stage? What are the family's strengths? How will you help the family manage their relative after discharge? In supervision, the resident's understanding of how family factors enhanced a particular treatment outcome or how a particular family interview was crucial in managing a patient within the family system can be discussed. Examples can be included in portfolios and case logs.

CASE EXAMPLE: ASSESSING A RESIDENT'S FAMILY SKILLS ON THE INPATIENT UNIT

Dr. Scott met with his adolescent patient, Anna, on the day of admission. Anna presented with symptoms of major depression and chronic pain. Her parents, she said, were forcing her to go to college and she couldn't tell them that she did not want to go because she was afraid they would throw her out of the house as they had her elder sister. Anna's father called Dr. Scott that evening and angrily peppered him with questions over the phone. The resident reassured him that his daughter was settling in well and had not been given any medication. He then scheduled a family meeting for the next morning to discuss the admission and proposed treatment. The following morning, Dr. Scott presented this new patient at rounds, citing family conflict as a contributing factor in the patient's illness. Dr. Scott indicated that a family meeting was urgently needed to assess the role of these family factors in the patient's condition, to provide the patient and family with psychoeducation about depression, and to discuss a proposed treatment plan. Dr. Scott mentioned that the father was angry and that it was important to find out what his concerns were.

At the family meeting, Dr. Scott listened to each family member's point of view, discussed the diagnosis, and encouraged family input into the treatment plan. The father was "against psychiatric drugs" because of what he had seen in the media. The mother agreed with the father. Dr. Scott, while respecting the family members' opinions, provided education about antidepressants, gave them literature to read, and encouraged them to call with any questions. He also indicated that they could attend the patient family psychoeducational group on the unit the following evening and gave them telephone numbers of community support groups. Dr. Scott and the family agreed that if Anna was not "better" in four days, they would agree to medication. The meeting was cordial and respectful, and the family expressed confidence that Dr. Scott had listened to and respected them.

After the meeting, the supervisor, who had been present during the meeting, reviewed Dr. Scott's family skills. The resident had identified the importance of family factors, reached out to the family, provided reassurance, and not pathologized the family. In addition, he had recognized the urgent need for a family intervention. The supervisor commended his ability to develop an alliance and trust with the family at this stage in treatment. The supervisor assessed Dr. Scott as having good family skills, proficient at level 3.

Residents report that the best learning experiences occur when they have involved supervision and cases in which a good outcome is likely (Guttman et al. 1999). Families who are overly anxious often are those for whom the onset of illness is a new experience or who have limited resources to care for a sick relative and are unable to take time off work to supervise their relative after discharge. These families also tend to lack understanding of the diagnostic process and the role of hospitalization. Especially in more challenging situations, the resident can best learn by first watching a senior clinician or psychiatrist interact with the family.

THE BENEFITS RESIDENTS REPORT FROM FAMILY-SKILLS TRAINING

According to a sample of former residents (from Massachusetts General Hospital and the University of Mississippi Medical Center, reported in Slovik et al. 1997), family skills are the tools least taught during residency and most needed after graduation. The most valuable skill these residents identified was a "systemic perspective" (i.e., the capacity to view clinical problems in a sociocultural context rather than as isolated phenomena). They also credited family skills, such as mapping genograms and prescribing behavioral assignments, with enabling them to be more active in other therapies. A minority of residents reported that overcoming their fear of meeting with more than one family member present at a time was a significant achievement! More than half of the residents recommended teaching of family skills early, in the second year of residency, citing family work as a good basis for the use of the biopsychosocial model (discussed in Chapter 2). Those who had learned family skills later in their training stated that it was difficult to shift from an individual approach to a systemic approach. The nontherapeutic settings in which these doctors used their family skills included negotiating with hospital administrators, supervising interdisciplinary teams, managing problems with office staff members, and supervising nonpsychiatric mental health professionals. Another surveyed group (from McGill University) reported similar opinions (Guttman et al. 1999). They also reported adopting a nonpathologizing approach to patients and learning how to develop interventions according to how patients and their families construct reality. One resident summed up family work this way: "It is not so much a tool as a way of looking at things."

Understanding how family systems work enables the clinician to bring a systems perspective to the interdisciplinary treatment team. There is often tension in an interdisciplinary team, as various members of the team may identify with different aspects of a patient. For example, the social worker may want the patient to be discharged as soon as possible, to care for children at home. The nurse is concerned about the patient's lack of understanding and laissez-faire attitude toward treatment and wants to prolong the hospital stay to provide further psychoeducation. The milieu therapist is suspicious that the patient is focusing too much on other patients and not engaging in her own treatment. The team leader can incorporate all these points of view into a systemic approach that is useful for the whole treatment team. In this case, the team leader hypothesizes that the patient's reluctance to engage in treatment is a way for her to avoid taking responsibility for her illness: by staying "sick" in the hospital, she is able to avoid the overwhelming responsibilities at home. The team as a whole can then strategize how best to help the patient. Each member of the team can have a specific role in helping the patient, while the team works together toward one goal. The social worker can focus on parenting needs, perhaps arranging parenting classes after discharge. The nurse can emphasize the importance of daily structure and help the patient decide the best time to take medications at home. The milieu therapist can redirect the patient to develop self-care skills for use when she feels overwhelmed at home. Thus, the team leader uses a systems perspective to ensure the optimal functioning of the treatment team.

SUMMARY

Comprehensive assessment of patients includes their families. The Accreditation Council for General Medical Education and the Group for the Advancement of Psychiatry's Committee on the Family have laid out how, in practice, residents can become competent at working with families. The ACGME has made it the responsibility of each residency program to implement these practices.

CHAPTER TWO

Biopsychosocial Case Formulation and Treatment Plan

This chapter discusses the biopsychosocial model, taking into account the latest research findings on the interaction between genetics and the environment. The limitations of the current use of the biopsychosocial model are discussed. A case example shows how family factors can be integrated into a biopsychosocial assessment and treatment plan.

Medical schools routinely teach medical students and residents about the biopsychosocial (BPS) model. Psychiatric residents are taught that they must ask about psychosocial factors and that treatment should take these factors into account. However, no direction is given as to *how* to integrate psychosocial factors into the assessment and treatment of patients. An inclusive, multiperspective model for psychiatric case formulation has been suggested (Weerasekera 1996) to facilitate the use of the BPS model, but the model has not been widely incorporated into psychiatric training.

A study of 33 residents from three different programs (McClain, O'Sullivan, and Clardy 2004) assessed residents' ability to provide a BPS case formulation. Residents were asked to complete a portfolio entry, which was to consist of the formulation itself, a self-reflective letter describing the rationale for selecting that particular case, and any relevant supporting documents, such as the initial psychiatric assessment and psychological testing. Residents were encouraged to select, from the cases they had managed within the previous academic year, the case that best demonstrated their ability to develop a BPS formulation. The description of the formulation to be created specified, "A biopsychosocial formulation requires the collection and synthesis of data in all these areas that leads to the formulation of a clear treatment plan," the case that "best demonstrates the complex interplay between the biological, psychological, social, and spiritual components of your patient's life" (p. 89). Nearly half of the residents reported either difficulty organizing the collected data into a formulation or difficulty doing so in a concise manner. Residents indicated that they needed to improve in their assessment of patients and needed more experience in formulating cases. Other residents reported that, when they formulated a case using the BPS model, their understanding of their patients increased and they had better supporting information for their diagnoses and treatment plans. Two trained raters, who were board-certified psychiatrists and not on the clinical faculty of any of the participating programs, stated that the most common problems for those residents who were rated as not competent were a "lack of integration" and a failure to recognize the interplay and impact each component of the BPS model had on the other components. This study indicates that, although the BPS formulation is generally accepted as an essential skill of practicing psychiatrists, some residents lack the ability to synthesize a coherent and succinct formulation.

Current psychiatric practice tends to consist of a biomedical assessment with an appended list of relevant psychosocial factors. In treatment, the psychiatrist using the biomedical model prescribes antidepressants and refers the patient to either a psychologist, who uses a cognitive-behavioral model and teaches cognitive strategies, or a social worker, who might use a systems model to attend to marital or social issues. This is described as "combined treatment," which Gabbard and Kay (2001) describe as "the essence of psychiatric practice and the most obvious example of the BPS foundation on which treatment decisions are based" (p. 1957). The current use of the term "BPS model" therefore connotes an additive treatment model that combines several treatments, with the expectation of producing a greater response than would a single-modality treatment. (For those who are interested, Keller et al. [2000], Luborsky et al. [1993], and Thase et al. [1997] provide good reviews of the evidence for the superiority of combined treatment over single treatment.) The popularity of additive treatment is bolstered by data that suggest that psychotherapy and pharmacotherapy work on different target symptoms and at different rates. Pharmacotherapy is thought to provide rapid, reliable relief from acute distress, and psychotherapy is thought to provide more enduring change (Hollon and Fawcett 1995). Combined treatment is described as enhancing the breadth, duration, and/or magnitude of the treatment response. However, it has been suggested that interactive and systems models are superior to the additive model and, in fact, George Engel had a systems model in mind when he created the BPS model.

ENGEL'S BIOPSYCHOSOCIAL MODEL

George Engel, in a celebrated lecture (1978), reflected on public criticism about the insensitivity of physicians. He attributed this attitude to medicine's focus on the biomedical model of disease and an inability to provide care, that is, to address the psychological and social aspects of illnesses. He stated, "Herein lies the dilemma. For while medicine recognizes the need to be more responsive to the growing public dissatisfaction with how individual care is being provided, the model upon which medical education and research is based does not include the patient. The biomedical model is disease-oriented, not patient-oriented. To be patient-oriented, the model must include psychosocial dimensions" (p. 171).

Engel advocated a systems-theoretical model for guiding medicine (1977). His BPS model is based on general systems theory (Bertalanffy 1968), which permits scientific investigation across different levels without attempting to reduce higher levels, as the reductionist biomedical model does. A systems model states, simply, that one part of the system affects another part and vice versa. Therefore, Engel suggested using this systems-theoretical framework to consider difficulties at the psychological, family, or social level along with the biomedical model and to work out how these factors might interact to produce disease. The BPS model replaced the simple cause-and-effect explanations of linear causality with a reciprocal causal model. Systems theory states that all levels of organization are linked to each other, so change in one level effects change in the other levels. Systems theory postulates that in a system there are "leading elements" that organize the other elements. The concept of the leading element is an important aspect of the systems model, and it is useful when assessing treatment options. The focus of a treatment intervention should, if possible, be on the leading element.

If the leading element is targeted, then other systemic changes follow more easily. However, it can be difficult to identify the leading element, and sometimes interventions at multiple points in the system are most effective, as in the additive model.

Philosophers and conceptual thinkers in psychiatry criticize the BPS model, saying that it perpetuates the dichotomy between the biological and the psychosocial, supports Cartesian dualism, and, at its most egregious, is the basis of the multiaxial DSM classification (Waterman 2005). From a historical perspective, Waterman continues, the BPS model was put forward in the 1980s to constrain the rise of biological psychiatry and to ensure that psychiatrists continue to take into account psychological factors and humanistic concerns when discussing psychiatric illnesses; however, the split between the biological and the psychosocial has been perpetuated. As our understanding of psychiatric illness becomes more sophisticated, particularly with the study of the environmental influences on gene expression, it is clear that the BPS model, as currently used, does not capture the many different levels of explanations about illnesses.

The BPS model is also accused of confusing etiology with treatment (Ghaemi 2003). For example, if an illness has psychological precipitants, it does not necessarily follow that the treatment should be psychological. Using the suppositions of the BPS model, as it is currently used, if family dysfunction or individual psychological dysfunction is found in the assessment, the finding dictates that treatment consist of family therapy or individual therapy. This is not necessarily the best approach; the use of medication to treat an underlying biological disorder may result in correction of the family or individual pathology; and paying attention to cultural factors may be crucial to allowing biological treatment to take place.

Other models have been suggested for describing psychiatric illnesses more accurately. The perspectives model discusses psychiatric illnesses from four perspectives: the concept of disease, dimensions of character, behaviors, and the concept of the life story (McHugh and Slavney 1998). A psychiatric illness usually falls into one of these four perspectives. Schizophrenia would be considered to fall into the disease perspective, personality disorder into the dimensions of character perspective, alcohol abuse into behaviors, and mild depression or anxiety into the concept of the life story.

The pluralistic model emphasizes that no single model can explain the entire range of psychiatric illnesses and that one should choose the best model for the situation at hand (Ghaemi 2003). Thus, a reductionist biological model is appropriate for biological research and a humanistic model is appropriate for dealing with questions about how to live one's life. A third model that has been put forward is the pragmatic model, which emphasizes evidenced-based treatments. It supports the use of multiple health care professionals, each providing treatment in his or her own area, rather than the use of one practitioner who is trained to a basic level in all modalities (Brendel 2005). Sadler (2005) suggests that ultimately, however, there may be no single overarching model for all aspects of psychiatry and we may have to live with the choice of different models.

From the perspective of the trainee, the BPS model has merit. It is easy to grasp, intuitive, and simple, a "good enough" working model, a folksy model that people, especially trainees, can bear in mind to refer to when assessing a patient and devising a treatment plan (Zacher 2005). If the BPS model acts as a reminder to assess patients fully and to consider all aspects of the patient when developing a treatment plan, then it has great utility. The American Board of Psychiatry and Neurology examiners for Part 2 expect psychiatric residents to develop a BPS case formulation and treatment plan. The expectation is that residents be able to describe biological and psychosocial etiological factors as well as to devise a treatment plan that consists of these elements.

HOW TO CONSTRUCT A BIOPSYCHOSOCIAL CASE FORMULATION AND TREATMENT PLAN

How can we use the BPS model to include family factors? Systems theory states that change in one part of a system affects the functioning of other parts of the system. This can be explained to the family as, "When one person is ill, the whole family is affected, and when the family is having difficulties, each family member will be affected." Using systems theory in family work means describing a problem by its effects on others, which in turn influences the problem. The following example illustrates how family factors are integrated into a BPS formulation and treatment plan.

CASE EXAMPLE: MR. AND MS. GREEN

Ms. Green is a 30-year-old, recently married woman, admitted with a diagnosis of recurrent major depression. She cannot sleep or eat, and she wishes she were dead. She thinks about taking an overdose of her medications. She has lost weight and is distraught and tearful at the initial interview, exclaiming that her marriage is over. Ms. Green has had three prior episodes of depression, the first when she was 17 years of age, and has been hospitalized on each occasion. She has worked part time and she lived with her parents until her marriage six months ago. Her mother has been very supportive of her throughout her previous episodes and, in fact, is the one who has now brought the patient to the hospital.

A meeting with the husband is scheduled for the morning after admission. At the meeting, it becomes clear that Ms. Green does not tell her husband when she becomes suicidal but instead goes to stay with her mother. Mr. Green says that is OK, because he doesn't know how to cope with his wife when she is suicidal. Mr. Green states that he does not want to get divorced and would like to help his wife but that he does not know what to do. He says he feels helpless and incompetent to help his wife. Ms. Green looks surprised and says she does not want to get divorced either but thought he did not care for her, as he turns away from her when she is ill.

The resident, Dr. Stevens, asks further questions about prodromal symptoms of Ms. Green's relapse and gently probes for ways in which Ms. and Mr. Green might recognize these symptoms when they start occurring and what Mr. Green could do that might be helpful. Ms. Green indicates that being in her husband's company is helpful. Mr. Green states that he does not know what to say to his wife when she is feeling unsafe. The two agree that when Ms. Green is feeling unsafe they could play a board game, something they enjoy. That way, they can be together without Mr. Green's being overwhelmed by fearing that he'll say the wrong thing. They work out a sequence of communication cues that they can use with each other so that the time spent together is supportive and not overwhelming. They agree on other cues to use when she needs to seek further help, such as an emergency visit to the outpatient treatment team. Both feel relieved at the end of the session, and another session is scheduled, to look at other aspects of their relationship.

In this case, there is clear demonstration of a transactional pattern in which Ms. Green's lack of communication leads to Mr. Green's withdrawal, which she interprets as a lack of caring and which reinforces her turning for support to her mother. The perceived loss of her husband's attention deepens her depression; she feels unlovable, and she feels hopeless about her marriage. Once this transactional pattern is brought out into the open and the couple clarify that the pattern is destructive and not what they want, they can actively work to change these behaviors. The focus in the follow-up session is on actions, such as spending time together, developing shared hobbies, and learning how to communicate effectively. The biological and family factors can be considered the leading elements in this system, and attention to these aspects leads to clinical improvement.

Case Formulation

The patient is a 30-year-old, recently married woman who presents with symptoms of major depression. She has had three prior episodes of depression, which have occurred at major transitions in her life and have responded well to a combination of pharmacotherapy and psychotherapy. The precipitating factor for the current episode is her recent marriage yet her continued reliance on her family of origin. There is a family history of depression in her paternal grandmother. There are no significant medical or substance abuse problems.

Treatment will consist of ecitalopram and a couples assessment to determine the viability of the patient's marriage. Couples therapy will be indicated, if the couple wishes to stay together. It is unclear at this time if the patient will require individual psychotherapy to reduce her reliance on her mother or whether that task can be accomplished as part of the couples therapy. Couples therapy will focus on improving communication and addressing early marital developmental issues. The short-term prognosis is good because the couple is motivated to participate in treatment together.

BIOPSYCHOSOCIAL RESEARCH

Only recently, as a result of research into the interaction between genes and the environment, have we begun to understand how biological and psychosocial/environmental factors interact to produce disease. Michael Rutter, one of the most eloquent researchers in this area, states, "Environments affect genes—not through effects on gene sequence, but through effects on gene expression. . . . Furthermore, environments affect neuroendocrine structure, and functioning, and through such effects, may influence brain development. Experiences may affect patterns of interpersonal interaction that become influential through their role in the shaping of later environments; in addition, experiences have to undergo cognitive and affective processing, so that what happens to individuals influences their mental concepts and models of themselves and their environments" (Rutter 2005, p. 5). What could more clearly describe the idea that George Engel had in mind when he devised the BPS model?

Two examples from current research support a gene/environment-interactive BPS model of disease. The first is a study of the relationship between biological (hormonal) factors and environmental (social support) factors in 160 women in the perinatal period (Ross, Sellers, et al. 2004). Depression and anxiety in the perinatal period are thought to be related to rapid changes in progesterone levels. In this study, variance in depressive symptoms was best accounted for by the indirect effects of biological risk factors (progesterone) on the psychosocial variable. The biological risk factor was thought to alter the sensitivity to the environmental stressor and thus to determine the threshold for the development of depressive and anxiety symptoms. This study supports a complex model in which biological and environmental factors interact to produce disease. This research does not describe a systems model of disease, as no transactional interaction is demonstrated. However, it can be categorized as an interactive model, integrating biological and psychosocial etiological factors in the production of disease.

The second example is adolescent conduct disorder. Research into this disorder is substantial, and researchers have tried to disentangle the genetic factors from the environmental factors, putting forward various disease models to explain how factors interrelate to produce this disorder. For many years, environmental factors were pitted against genetic factors, but most contemporary theories acknowledge the importance of each factor as well as the importance of their interaction. The major question has become how these factors relate to each other to produce conduct disorder. Several different models are proposed to explain conduct disorder (Dodge and Pettit

2003). The simplest is an additive model that describes a degree of risk that is linearly related to the number of risk factors present. In this model, the odds of the disorder's occurring are increased by the addition of risk factors. Interactive models describe a process whereby certain risk factors exert influence only in the presence (or absence) of other risk factors. For example, it may be that some life experiences lead to conduct disorder only when they occur in children who are initially biologically predisposed to the disorder. Systems models describe nonlinear processes in which the child and the social environment interact in a dynamic way to lead to conduct disorder. A transactional developmental model leads to an understanding of how multiple factors unfold over time.

According to Rutter (2005), environmental, genetic, and developmental perspectives in an integrated model best describe the pathways to conduct disorder. His theoretical model is complex and is derived from the evidence provided by many studies over the past several decades. Children with certain genetic predispositions are likely to elicit particular reactions from parents and peers. A child who is temperamentally fussy may lead his or her parents to respond with harsh discipline. The child may bring on rejection by peers by behaving in ways that peers find unacceptable. Other factors, such as poverty, also influence parenting. Over time, parenting, peer experiences, and social experiences alter the child's biological dispositions. Thus, children are born with biological dispositions or into sociocultural contexts that launch them on a trajectory toward conduct problems in later life. These factors tend to direct a child toward particular life experiences, such as harsh discipline or emotional neglect or conflict with peers and siblings. Eventually, the child acquires relational schemas made up of hostility, aggression, and self-defensive goals. Thus, when confronted with problematic social situations, these children readily make hostile attributions about peers and adults and act aggressively without thinking about consequences. The environment then usually reacts to them with hostility and punishment, and a vicious cycle ensues. This transactional developmental model coincides with Engel's BPS model.

The next chapter describes family research in detail, but two studies on families will be cited here to provide further evidence for the utility of the BPS model: Adoptees at high genetic risk for schizophrenic spectrum disorders are significantly more sensitive to adverse rearing patterns in their adoptive families than are adoptees without this genetic risk (Tienari et al. 2004). Also, maladaptive parental behavior, not psychiatric illness, is associated with an increased risk in the offspring for anxiety, depression, disruptive personality, and substance abuse disorders during late adolescence and early adulthood (Johnson et al. 2001). The number of offspring with conduct disorder increases markedly as the number of maladaptive parental behaviors increases. The BPS model is therefore evolving into a model that can accurately reflect the latest gene/environmental research, as well as being useful as a working model for clinicians when thinking about the patient and the environment.

SUMMARY

The biopsychosocial model serves to ensure that all aspects of the patient and his or her environment are considered in assessment and treatment. Recent sophisticated research has demonstrated how biological and psychosocial factors interrelate in both the etiology and the course of psychiatric illnesses. The resident who is fully informed about biopsychosocial research is well prepared to deliver optimal care and to make recommendations regarding effective treatment.

PART TWO

Research on Families and Family Treatments

CHAPTER THREE

Research on Families

This chapter reviews research on the influence of families in both general medicine and psychiatry. Studies of family factors are spread across many disciplines and are not immediately accessible to someone interested in the breadth and depth of family research. This chapter brings together these research findings to inform our understanding of the role of family in psychiatric illnesses and treatments. It presents knowledge of family research that can satisfy the family component of the psychiatry core competencies.

The influence of family on disease and treatment can be studied in many ways. Most simply, family factors are studied as variables in the disease process—for example, a study might assess the effect of family support on the outcome of a disease. More sophisticated family studies examine how family processes mediate between risk variables in the expression of disease. Three areas of family research are given prominence in this chapter: family resilience, the interaction between genetics and the environment, and expressed emotion. Following this discussion, family research in general medicine and specific psychiatric disorders is presented.

FAMILY RESILIENCE

After decades of looking at critical and dysfunctional families, researchers are now turning their attention to the study of family strengths. Family strengths can be conceptualized as simple protective factors, such as the presence of social support. Family resilience, however, implies that a family has a specific internal organization or has reorganized in a specific way to protect against stress. The degree of resilience present in a family may become known only when the family is exposed to a stress, such as coping with illness. Resilience is conceptualized as the interplay of multiple risk and protective family processes that occur over time, and it involves individual, family, and other sociocultural influences (Garmezy 1991).

One study of 700 people born in 1955 illustrates how family strengths influence individual outcome over time. Seven hundred children of plantation workers living in poverty in Hawaii were followed for forty years (Werner 1993). By age 18, two-thirds of the children had done poorly in terms of emotional development but one-third had developed into competent, caring, and confident young adults. Through midlife, all but two of these competent adults were still living successful lives. All of the competent adults had had significant relationships with family members, partners, adult mentors, or teachers. These significant "family" relationships were thought to act as mediating protective factors that positively influenced the trajectory of these individuals' lives as children, resulting in resilient adults.

What specific family processes contribute to family resilience? Several constructs have been considered by researchers, such as a sense of family coherence (Antonovsky 1987) and the ability to stay connected (Beavers and Hampson 1990). Clear and direct communication and collaborative problem solving are other factors identified as important healthy family processes (Ryan et al. 2005). Many family members report resilience developed from coping with mental illness. In one study, 87.7 percent of families who had dealt with a family member's mental illness reported family resilience and 99.2 percent of family members reported personal resilience (Lefley 1992). One family member in this study stated, "When a family experiences something like this, it makes for very compassionate people—people of substance. My brother created a bond among us that we will not allow to be broken" (Marsh and Lefley 1996, p. 4). Families in Marsh and Lefley's 1996 study had the following suggestions for psychiatrists, to help them foster this kind of resilience:

1. Professionals should use competency-based models rather than pathology-based models; the latter foster dependency and learned helplessness and undermine self-esteem.

2. Professionals should work with families to establish partnerships that promote an atmosphere of mutual respect; respect the needs, desires, and concerns of families; include families in decisions that involve them; and develop mutual goals for treatment and rehabilitation.

3. Professionals should acknowledge the needs of families and teach them skills to cope with the illness.

4. Professionals should recognize the potential for resilience among family members, encourage resilient thinking and behavior, and reinforce resilience when it occurs. This stance will counter the adverse effects of earlier models that pathologized and disempowered families.

GENETICS AND THE FAMILY ENVIRONMENT

The expectation that a direct link exists between gene and disease has not proven true for psychiatric disorders. There is, however, clear interdependency between genetic and environmental influences on disease, with biological factors affecting the expression of disease only in the presence of certain environmental stressors. Adoption and twin studies help tease out the relative influence of genetic and environmental factors. Schizophrenia and conduct disorder are two areas of research on the interaction between genetics and the environment.

Finnish investigators found that adoptees at high genetic risk for schizophrenia-spectrum disorders are more sensitive to adverse rearing patterns in their adoptive families than are adoptees without this genetic risk (Tienari et al. 2004). In this longitudinal study, adopted-away offspring of mothers with diagnoses of schizophrenia-spectrum disorders were compared with adopted-away offspring of biological mothers without schizophrenia-spectrum diagnoses. The adoptees at low genetic risk had biological mothers with either a non–schizophrenia-spectrum psychiatric diagnosis or no psychiatric diagnosis. Experienced psychiatrists evaluated the family environments of the adoptive parents, using tape recordings made over 14–16 hours. They conducted joint interviews with the whole family and with the parental couples as well as semistructured personal interviews with individual family members. Three domains of family functioning were identified as being associated with unhealthy rearing practices: "critical/conflictual," "constricted," and "boundary problems." Only in the adoptees at high genetic risk was there a significant association between a diagnosis of schizophrenia-spectrum disorder and adverse rearing patterns. This can be interpreted as an example of interaction between genotype and the environment; that is, adoptees at genetic risk are more sensitive to problems in the adoptive family.

Conduct disorder, a second area of research on the interaction between genetics and the environment, is difficult to study because there are so many variables to untangle and the disease unfolds slowly over time. Conduct disorder is known to "run in families." Does this mean that parental behavior causes conduct disorder, or does it mean that an inherited gene(s) causes conduct disorder? Researchers have argued for decades about the relative merits of these two positions, usually settling for a model that includes multiple factors.

Maladaptive parenting has long been viewed as an important determinant of childhood psychopathology. Maladaptive parenting includes inconsistent enforcement of rules, loud arguments between the parents, difficulty controlling anger toward the child, maternal possessiveness, use of guilt to control the child, and verbal abuse. The relationship between parenting and psychiatric disorders was assessed in a longitudinal study that conducted evaluations of 593 biological parents and their offspring from 1975 to 1993. In 1975, the offspring had a mean age of 6 years. Maladaptive parental behavior (not psychiatric illness) was associated with an increased risk in the offspring for anxiety, depression, disruptive personality, and substance use disorders during late adolescence and early adulthood (Johnson et al. 2001). All of these associations remained significant after parental psychiatric disorders were controlled for statistically. The number of offspring with conduct disorder increased markedly as the number of maladaptive parental behaviors increased. In conclusion, children of parents with psychiatric disorders are at increased risk for psychiatric disorders only if there is a history of maladaptive parental behavior.

Looking more specifically at conduct disorder, antisocial behavior is associated with biological variance, such as low MAO-A activity. Maltreated boys with a variant of the MAO-A gene that produces low MAO-A activity are more likely to develop antisocial behavior than are boys with the variant of the MAO-A gene that produces high MAO-A activity (Caspi et al. 2002). However, the low-activity MAO-A gene has been found to be a risk factor only when combined with an adverse childhood environment, such as inconsistent parental discipline, parental neglect, or exposure to interparental violence (Foley et al. 2004).

In studies of twin registries and of other adoption programs for which family history is available, the relative influences on children can be divided into genetic, shared environmental, and nonshared environmental influences (Reiss et al. 2001). The results of the research into relative influence are complex, but a few pertinent findings can be described. Adopted children at genetic risk for antisocial behavior are more likely to receive negative parenting from their adoptive parents than are children not at genetic risk (O'Connor et al. 1998). However, the researchers state that most of the association is not explicable on the basis of a correlation between genetics and the environment and that an additional environmental effect on the children's behavior is influential. Influences unique to each sibling in a twin pair also account for some variance (Reiss et al. 1995). Conflictual and negative parental behavior directed specifically at an adolescent was found to be responsible for 60 percent of the variance in adolescent antisocial behavior (Reiss et al. 2001). Moreover, harsh parental behavior directed at one sibling can have a protective effect on the other sibling, a phenomenon called the "sibling barricade." In Reiss's research on antisocial behavior, the influence of nonshared experiences is more important than genetic influences.

Why are these findings important for psychiatrists? In essence, research reveals that, for complex diseases, the family environment plays a significant role in protecting family members or placing them at risk. Furthermore, the family environment can be seen as consisting of distal risks and proximal risks (Rutter 2005). Distal risks include such factors as poverty, which makes good parenting more difficult. Proximal risks consist of the immediate dysfunctional family environment. Expressed emotion is one such characteristic of the immediate family environment that can be considered a proximal risk.

EXPRESSED EMOTION

Expressed emotion (EE), a construct that has been around for more than 40 years, measures criticism, hostility, and emotional overinvolvement. The expressed emotion construct originated when George Brown and colleagues at the Social Research Unit in London explored the role of environmental factors in the prognosis of patients with schizophrenia. They found that patients were more likely to relapse if they returned to live with parents or spouses than if they went to live in lodgings or with siblings (Brown, Carstairs, and Topping 1958). They hypothesized that the close emotional ties of family life overstimulated the patients with schizophrenia, and they thought the patients became withdrawn and isolated in an attempt to reduce their level of social contact.

What exactly is EE? Researchers assessing the components of the family environment created scales for measuring criticism, hostility, emotional overinvolvement (EOI), warmth, and positive comments. EE measures the number of critical and positive comments made during a family interview. Criticisms are defined as comments about the behavior or characteristics of the patient which the respondent clearly resents or is annoyed by. Hostility is rated categorically, according to whether the respondent makes generalized criticisms of the patient, expresses attitudes that are rejecting of the patient, neither of these, or both. Scores for EOI and warmth are assigned by the rater after taking into account comments made and attitudes expressed throughout the interview. The EOI score represents a composite measure of factors such as an exaggerated emotional response, overintrusive or self-sacrificing behavior, and overidentification with the patient. Warmth is rated on a six-point scale. These scales became the family construct called EE, assessed using a structured interview called the Camberwell Family Interview. Although initially used with schizophrenic patients and their families, EE is now studied extensively across the health care spectrum and in many cultures (Wearden et al. 2000).

Initially, EE was considered to be static (Leff and Vaughn 1985). Low EE relatives were described as tolerant, nonintrusive, and sensitive to the patient's needs, while high EE relatives were described as intolerant of the patient's problems, intrusive, and making use of inappropriate and inflexible strategies to cope with difficulties. However, this static conceptualization has proven too simplistic, and current studies of EE reveal that it measures a much more fluid process—the internal components of the EE in a patient's environment change over time. In a study of first- or early-admission psychotic patients and their relatives that followed the subjects for 18 months, a relationship between high EE and relapse was found; but the internal components of the EE to which the patient was exposed changed during the study period. Overinvolvement predominated at the initial evaluation but marked criticism had superseded it at 18 months (Stirling et al. 1993). Family members were overly involved with their relative when the illness began, but as the illness progressed, criticism predominated. High EE in families can also result from ongoing stressful interaction with a disturbed family member, thus indicating a bidirectional process (Miklowitz 2004). This suggests that EE measures a dynamic process and that family attitudes may evolve during the course of a relative's illness. EE appears to be not a family trait, as was originally thought, but rather a reflection of family processes that change over time.

Can EE be assessed easily? Measuring a family's level of EE using the Camberwell Family Interview requires training, and the interview takes 1–2 hours to administer (Vaughn and Leff 1976a). EE can also be measured using the five-minute speech sample (Magana et al. 1986). A high score on criticism is given if a family member makes a negative initial statement, gives a negative relationship rating, or makes one or more critical comments. A high EOI score is given if during the interview there is self-sacrificing or overprotective behavior, emotional display, or any two of the following are made: (1) recounting of excessive detail about the past, (2) one or more statements of attitude, or (3) excessive praise (five or more positive remarks). The five-minute speech sample is indicative of borderline high EE if the family member expresses dissatisfaction with the patient. In clinical use, say Hooley and Teasdale (1989), one question is likely to reveal a high EE. If you have only one question to ask a patient about the family, ask, "How critical is your [family member] of you?" If the patient says, "Very critical," EE can be suspected to be high.

How do families with high EE scores behave? The example of families of people with schizophrenia is illustrative. Relatives with high EE appear to be more controlling of their ill relative, possibly thinking that their relative cannot take care of him- or herself (Hooley and Campbell 2002). High EE relatives most commonly believe that the abnormal behavior of the patient, especially negative behavior, is under the patient's control; they will say, "He's just lazy" (Brewin et al. 1991). Family members who judge the patient as responsible for his or her own behavior will feel angry and annoyed when the patient shows symptoms such as social withdrawal. Family members who judge the patient as not responsible for his or her behavior will tend to feel sympathetic and concerned. Attributing the problem behaviors as internal to and controllable by the patient may lead relatives to coerce the patient "to get back to normal." This can then become a critical attitude in which family members become angry at the patient's willfulness and refusal to try. Relatives who understand the patient's behavior to be symptomatic of schizophrenia have lower EE and are much less critical of the patient. Also, when family members are working outside the home, the family tends to have lower EE, suggesting that the working family members are less involved and more focused on their own lives (Scazufca and Kuipers 1996). Looking at attributions (i.e., how the family members understand the cause of the patient's symptoms) has become an important new direction in family research. In fact, attributional variables are statistically more reliable predictors of schizophrenia relapse at nine months follow-up than are EE measures, supporting the idea that relatives' cognitions are of primary importance to the link between EE and relapse (Barrowclough and Hooley 2003).

However, the EE construct again confounds us. The attributions made by family members who are designated as emotionally overinvolved are different from the attributions of other high EE family members (Barrowclough, Johnston, and Tarrier 1994; Brewin et al. 1991). EOI family members may perceive their ill relative as not responsible for his or her own behavior; thus, the patient is seen as incompetent and the family then takes over and does everything for the patient. Based on the level of EOI, EE is high even though criticism is low. So, measures of EE for two families can be high but the internal components that create the high rating can differ.

The recent interest in resilience has highlighted another problem with research on EE: the positive components originally included in the measure (Brown and Rutter 1966) had come to be ignored, so EE measures had been portraying families in a negative light, blaming high EE family members for their ill relatives' relapses. Recently, the concept of family warmth has been resurrected as a focus of family research (Barrowclough, Johnston, and Tarrier 1994). It has been reported that relapse is less likely when patients with schizophrenia return to households high in warmth than when they return to households low in warmth (Bertrando et al. 1992; Ivanović, Vuletić, and Bebbington 1994). Patients whose relatives show warmth without criticism or overinvolvement have a significantly better outcome.

EE also varies across cultures (Jenkins and Karno 1992). Patients with schizophrenia in developing countries have a better prognosis than do patients in developed countries (Thara 2004). Does the family environment have anything to do with this difference? Could the family environment be less critical (lower EE) in developing countries, resulting in a better outcome for these patients? Of all ethnic groups, European Americans are documented to have the highest ratings of EE. It was found that 67 percent of Anglo-American families residing in southern California can be designated as high EE (Vaughn et al. 1984); among Caucasian Canadians the proportion is 61 percent (King and Dixon 1999). High EE ratings are found in 41 percent of Mexican American families (Karno et al. 1987), and 45 percent of British families fall into the category (Vaughn and Leff 1976b). India has the lowest percentage of high EE families—only 23 percent (Leff et al. 1987). However, the significance of EE varies across cultures. There is no difference in relapse rates for schizophrenia for patients living in high EE families and low EE families in Iran, where high EE is found in 60 percent of families (Mottaghipour et al. 2001), nor in China, where high EE is found in 42 percent of families (Phillips and Xiang 1995). In Egypt, where high EE is found in 55 percent of families, patients with schizophrenia tolerate higher levels of criticism before relapse than do patients in the West (Kamal 1995). In Japan, however, high EE, which is present in 58 percent of households, is associated with high relapse rates (Tanaka, Mino, and Inoue 1995).

Emotional overinvolvement is the EE component whose influence is most likely to vary across cultures (Bhugra and McKenzie 2003). In sociocentric societies, emotional overinvolvement is to be expected, because the individual is seen as part of a close-knit family group. In Indian families and in Jewish families, it is culturally acceptable for mothers to be overly involved with their sons and it is not considered pathological. However, changes in EE occur as individuals and families migrate, and measures of EE may be difficult to interpret in families who are partially acculturated or of mixed ethnicity. Unexpected findings continue to surface in research on EE. Family warmth serves as a protective factor in the course of illness for Mexican Americans who return to households identified as high in family warmth, but for Anglo-American families, family warmth seems not to influence the course of illness (Kopelowicz et al. 2002; López et al. 2004). Consistent with prior research, family criticism predicts relapse for Anglo-American patients. Thus, the role of the family in schizophrenia differs for Mexican American and Anglo-American patients. It is clear that the emotional environment within which patients live can have profound effects on the course of their illness, however, it is not clear if EE is a useful measure cross-culturally.

In summary, whatever the construct of EE is measuring, high EE in most places is considered a significant and robust predictor of relapse in many psychiatric illnesses (Butzlaff and Hooley 1998), including schizophrenia (Kavanaugh 1992), depressive disorders (Hooley and Teasdale 1989), acute mania (Miklowitz and Goldstein 1997), and alcoholism (O'Farrell et al. 1998).

GENERAL MEDICINE

The family provides an intimate and emotionally intense relationship that persists over time, and the quality of that relationship can have a significant influence on outcome for patients with many diseases. Research about the role of families in general medicine focuses mostly on chronic illness. Campbell (2003) makes four statements about how family factors influence the course and outcome of chronic illnesses: (1) the power of families' influence on health equals that of traditional medical risk factors; (2) for adults, marriage is the family relationship that most influences health; (3) emotional support is the most important and influential type of support provided by families; and (4) negative, critical, or hostile family relationships have a stronger influence on health than do positive or supportive relationships.

Several research examples of the effect of emotional support can be found. For example, women with cardiovascular disease who receive positive family support have a better outcome than do women who do not receive positive family support (Coyne et al. 2001), and emotional support improves the outcome of hospitalized elderly patients with acute myocardial infarction at six months follow-up (Berkman, Leo-Summers, and Horwitz 1992). More sophisticated studies examine *how* family processes influence the expression of disease. For instance, it has been determined that some dysfunctional family processes may have their origin in the stresses and strains of caring for an ill family member, referred to as the caregiver burden. The multiple changes that families undergo when someone in the family has a chronic illness are well described (Rolland 1994), and the demands of caregiving can exact an emotional toll as well as impose effects on the family's organization, communication, and goals (Heru 2000). The whole family may need to reorganize, and life goals may need to be changed. For most chronic illnesses, the family's ability to provide consistent management is crucial for optimal outcome.

Family factors can be classified as protective factors or risk factors. Five general protective factors and six general risk factors were identified in a review of the literature (Weihs, Fisher, and Baird 2002) (Table 3.1). Protective factors include healthy family processes, such as good coping skills that do not allow the disease to interfere with normal family developmental tasks. Healthy families are characterized as communicating well, encouraging individual family members, expressing appreciation, being committed to the family, having a religious or spiritual orientation, being part of a larger social group, being adaptable, having clear roles, and spending time together (Stinnett and DeFrain 1985; Krysan, Moore, and Zill 1990). Importantly, family strengths can mitigate family weaknesses. For example, good parenting can offset family difficulties in the healthy development of children (Luthar, Cicchetti, and Becker 2000).

Family risk factors include intrafamilial conflict, blame, rigidity, and high levels of criticism. The strong negative effect of criticalness and hostility on the outcome of disease was emphasized in Campbell's and Weihs's literature reviews. Caregiving can also be considered a family risk factor. Caregivers report more general health problems, including influenza, upper respiratory infections, stomach disorders, headaches, back pain, sleeplessness, and depression than similar populations who do not experience caregiver burden (National Family Caregivers Association 1997). A specific example is that women who care for a disabled or ill spouse for nine or more hours per

TABLE 3.1
Risk and Protective Family Factors

Protective Factors	Risk Factors
Clear family organization	Perfectionism and rigidity
Family connectedness	Intrafamilial conflict
Mutually supportive family relationships	Criticism or blame
	External stress
Direct communication about the illness and its management	Interruption of family members' developmental tasks by disease
Caregiver coping skills	Psychological trauma related to diagnosis and treatment of disease

Source: Adapted from Weihs, Fisher, and Baird 2002.

TABLE 3.2
Possible Protective Family Factors

Ease and comfort with direct communication about personal issues

Emotional expressiveness with little avoidance of emotional issues and little use of guilt

Moderate to high levels of emotional involvement

Secure attachments

Tolerance of repetition, ritual, and routine

Integration of rituals and routines into family life

Family time for recreation

Problem-solving capacity

Congruence within the family of beliefs about health and disease

Families able to invest in disease management and conjointly acknowledge the disease

Family adjustment to diagnosis predicts family adjustment to disease management

Alliance between patient and health care provider

Source: Adapted from Weihs, Fisher, and Baird 2002.

week are at increased risk of coronary artery disease (Lee et al. 2003). Some high-risk family factors are not malleable, such as low socioeconomic status and patient and family pre-illness psychopathology. These risk factors can be used, however, to identify patients and families at high risk and to target these patients and families for selective interventions. Many risk factors are malleable, however, and providing family intervention to mitigate them has been studied as a way to improve health care outcomes (see Chapter 4).

A dozen factors that may be protective have also been identified (Table 3.2), but there is not sufficient evidence to confirm their beneficial effect on the outcome of disease. They include, for example, being able to talk about emotional issues and the integration of ritual and routine in family life. Secure attachments, good problem-solving ability, and having family recreation time are other potentially protective factors. If these factors are addressed in treatment, they will result, at the very least, in a greater sense of well-being in the family.

PSYCHIATRY

When the families of psychiatric inpatients are assessed, dysfunction is found across all psychiatric diagnostic groups. Among families of inpatients,

patients with major depression, alcohol dependence, and adjustment disorders are reported to have the poorest family functioning (Miller et al. 1986). It is unclear if family dysfunction occurs because of the disruption of hospitalization and/or the disease or if the family dysfunction is a factor in the illness or plays a role in the need for hospitalization. Whatever the case, these findings point to the need to understand the families of inpatients.

Schizophrenia

Twenty years ago, the debate about the etiology of schizophrenia focused on the influence of "nature versus nurture." Current research is examining the interaction between nature and nurture, and plenty of evidence is being found. As described above, children at high genetic risk for schizophrenia are more sensitive to problems in childrearing, and patients in high EE families have relapse rates three to four times greater than those in low EE families at the nine-month follow-up (Parker and Hadzi-Pavlovic 1990).

In addition, the course of schizophrenia is affected by cultural practices. For example, 75–85 percent of Latino patients with schizophrenia live with their families, compared to 66 percent of African American patients and 40 percent of European American patients (Guarnaccia and Parra 1996; Jenkins and Schumacher 1999). White American caregivers of adults with schizophrenia report higher levels of burden and lower levels of caregiver satisfaction than African American caregiving mothers, despite the fact that the white Americans are healthier, wealthier, more educated, and have more spousal support (Pruchno, Patrick, and Burant 1997). The role of socioeconomic status, life expectations, and attitudes toward mental illness may account for these differences.

Bipolar Disorder

Patients with bipolar disorder relapse at higher rates if they live with high EE relatives (Miklowitz et al. 1988; Okasha et al. 1994). A relapse rate *eight times* greater was found at the nine-month follow-up for patients who returned to high EE families than for those who did not (Priebe, Wildgrube, and Muller-Oerlinghausen 1989). Patients with bipolar disorder who live with high EE relatives are five times more likely to experience a depressive recurrence than patients with low EE relatives (Yan et al. 2004). The study by Yan and colleagues demonstrated polarity-specific effects of high EE on recurrence in bipolar disorder. Negative life events and poor social support are also known to be associated with more depressive symptoms and recurrences, compared to manic episodes (Cohen et al. 2004; Gitlin et al. 1995; Johnson and Kizer 2002; Johnson et al. 1999). Perhaps depressive episodes are more influenced by psychosocial variables than are manic episodes.

A recent study of families of patients with bipolar disorder attempted to link three concepts: caregiver burden, emotional overinvolvement, and patient outcome. Families who experienced the highest burden in caring for their relative also showed the highest EOI. The patients in these families had poor adherence to their medication regimens, resulting in an increased likelihood of relapse (Perlick et al. 2004). Neither the severity of symptoms nor whether or not they lived with the patient affected the family members' experience of burden. However, burden was significantly associated with the family's perception of stigma regarding psychiatric illness. This study is an example of biopsychosocial research that shows social attitudes affecting family behavior and family behavior in turn influencing the patient's behavior, resulting in a change in the patient's outcome.

Major Depression

Patients have a slower rate of recovery from a major depressive episode when they live in families with significant family dysfunction (Keitner and Miller 1990; Miller et al. 1992). Patients with good family functioning at the time of hospitalization generally maintain their healthy functioning after discharge and are more likely to recover by 12 months than are patients with poor family functioning (Keitner et al. 1995). Good family functioning is described as one of five factors that improve outcome in major depression (Keitner et al. 1992).

Patients with major depression also show high relapse rates and relapse at relatively low levels of criticism when they live with high EE relatives (Hooley, Orley, and Teasdale 1986). Two or more critical comments, during the Camberwell Family Interview, are associated with relapse for patients with major depression, compared to six or more critical comments for patients with schizophrenia (Vaughn and Leff 1976a). Typically, family members of patients with major depression make at least seven, and often more than eight, critical remarks (Hooley, Orley, and Teasdale 1986; Vaughn and Leff 1976a). These families would certainly be classified as high EE. Lower ratings of EE are found when the patient is elderly, with only four to five critical comments, and the highest ratings occur in patients who have recurrent or chronic illnesses (Hinrichsen, Adelstein, and McMeniman 2004). Having a partner who is consistently uncritical or who is critical only at presentation is associated with the best prognosis for major depression (Hayhurst et al. 1997).

Obsessive-Compulsive Disorder

Children with obsessive-compulsive disorder (OCD) often live in families with high EE (Hibbs et al. 1991), low emotional support, and low warmth and closeness (Valleni-Basile et al. 1995). These families use few good problem-solving techniques and reward these children less for independent behavior (Barrett, Shortt, and Healy 2002). When parents become involved in the child's OCD rituals, there is increased family distress, marital discord, and sibling problems (Barrett, Rasmussen, and Healy 2001). Greater accommodation by family members to OCD behaviors causes more family dysfunction, increases family stress, and promotes more frequent rejecting attitudes toward the patient (Steketee and Van Noppen 2003). Accommodation to OCD behavior by family members includes providing reassurance that the behavior is acceptable, actively participating in rituals and/or avoidance at the patient's request, taking over the patient's duties, and modifying family activities and routines to accommodate the patient's obsessive-compulsive symptoms. Thus, reducing EE and reducing accommodation to the OCD behaviors results in better outcomes for the children.

Alcohol Abuse and Dependence

In the past, spouses of alcoholic persons were pathologized and blamed for enabling the patient's drinking. Wives of alcoholic men were thought to possess personality traits that caused them to exhibit irrational enabling behaviors. Thankfully, this view has been replaced with the belief that enabling behaviors are normal reactions to the stress in an alcohol-involved family. Enabling behaviors are now described as learned behaviors that influence the patient's drinking or drug-using behaviors, through either positive or negative reinforcement, and that increase the probability of recurrence. These enabling behaviors include lying or making excuses to family or friends (69% of spouses do this), performing the patient's neglected chores (69%), threatening separation but not following through (67%), changing or canceling family plans or social activities because of the drinking or drug use (49%), making excuses for the patient's impaired behavior (44%), giving money to the patient to buy alcohol or drinking in the patient's presence (30%), and purchasing alcohol or drugs for the patient (22%) (Rotunda, West, and O'Farrell 2004). These unintentionally enabling partners, although indulging in these behaviors, declared abstinence to be their goal for the abuser. Regarding the influence of EE, alcoholic patients are more likely to relapse, to relapse sooner, and to drink on a greater percentage of days if they have high EE spouses rather than low EE spouses. EE remains associated with relapse even when the results are adjusted for patients' age, education, and severity of alcohol problem (O'Farrell et al. 1998).

Other Illnesses

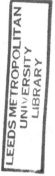

Intensity of expressed emotion in family members affects prognosis in many other psychiatric illnesses. For patients with eating disorders and obesity, for example, high EE is a strong predictor of poor outcome (van Furth et al. 1996). On the other hand, high levels of emotional overinvolvement are associated with a lower probability of hospital readmissions among patients with borderline personality disorder after 12 months (Hooley and Hoffman 1999). This finding can be explained by the extreme sensitivity to rejection of persons with borderline personality disorder.

SUMMARY

Family factors have been widely researched in general medicine and psychiatry. Research on expressed emotion and on genetics has been conducted for many decades and provides substantial evidence for the role of family factors in the onset and course of psychiatric illness. Research continues to unravel the complexities of expressed emotion and attempts to understand how some family processes contribute to family resilience. Perhaps the research of most importance is the longitudinal research on the interaction between genetics and the environment that categorically places family factors at the genesis of many complex illnesses. The depth and breadth of knowledge concerning the role of family factors in medical and psychiatric illnesses clearly justifies the importance of understanding family factors in psychiatry.

CHAPTER FOUR

Family Treatments

Family-based treatment interventions are a significant contribution to psychiatric practice. Many randomized clinical trials have demonstrated that family-based interventions reduce relapse rates, improve recovery, and improve family well-being among participants. This chapter gives an overview of research into family-based treatment of medical and psychiatric illnesses. The current American Psychiatric Association Practice Guidelines are reviewed.

The inpatient psychiatrist needs to understand the breadth and depth of family interventions. The first part of this chapter outlines research on family interventions in general medicine, in disciplines other than psychiatry. The family-based treatments in psychiatry that are most relevant for the inpatient psychiatrist are reviewed in the next section, then applications to individual disorders are discussed. The American Psychiatric Association's Practice Guidelines recommendations regarding family-based interventions are outlined.

GENERAL MEDICINE

Most research on family-based interventions is conducted with children and elderly persons. These two populations are usually dependent on other family members for help with the management of illness, so family members are often involved in their care. As discussed in Chapter 3, many illnesses are significantly influenced, positively or negatively, by family factors, thus highlighting the importance of including the family in assessment and in the planning of treatment, particularly for chronic illnesses. Family intervention studies in general medicine fall into four main subject areas: childhood chronic illnesses, spousal involvement in chronic adult illnesses, family caregiving of elders, and health promotion and disease prevention (Campbell 2003). This section will give two examples of research from the general medicine literature supporting the efficacy of family interventions.

In diabetes, successful family involvement in treatment preserves health and prevents long-term complications. Researchers at the Joslin Diabetes Center in Boston (Laffel et al. 2003) developed a low-cost intervention to reduce family conflict in the management of diabetes in adolescents. One hundred and five children and adolescents, aged from 8 to 17 years, who had had insulin-dependent diabetes for at least 6 years, were randomly assigned to receive a family-focused intervention or standard multidisciplinary diabetes care. Patients in both groups were seen at 3- to 4-month intervals and were followed prospectively for a year. The two groups had the same number of visits (4.6 at 1-year follow-up) and received the same educational materials about diabetes. The family-focused intervention group received further instruction: on ways to set goals, on identifying tasks regarding diabetes health maintenance, and on effective problem solving of diabetes-related concerns. The family-focused group emphasized teamwork, particularly in the area of insulin injections and measurement of blood glucose. Furthermore, at each visit one of four instruction modules was implemented: (1) spoken communication about diabetes, (2) review of educational material pertaining to the disease, (3) encouraging family discussion regarding elevated blood sugar, and (4) facilitating use of a log book to deal with out-of-range blood sugar values. The implementation of this family intervention with adolescents was found to significantly improve management of the illness and of family relationships and to prevent complications, at little added expense to the clinic.

The second example concerns adults with systemic lupus erythematosus (SLE). Good self-care skills, good partner support, and good problem-solving skills have been shown to result in better outcomes for adults with SLE. Sixty-four adults with SLE and their partners received psychoeducational instruction geared to enhancing self-efficacy, couple communication about the disease, social support, and problem solving. The instruction consisted of a one-hour session with a nurse educator, followed by monthly counseling by telephone for six months. A control group of 55 patients and their partners received an attention placebo consisting of a 45-minute video presentation about lupus and monthly telephone follow-up calls for six months. After one year, the group receiving psychoeducation reported improved communication, increased levels of social support, and reduced levels of patient fatigue, compared to the control group (Karlson et al. 2004). This research provides an example of improved patient outcomes through the modification of family risk factors (as discussed in Chapter 3).

An effective family-focused approach to the management of chronic disease should address three main goals (Weihs, Fisher, and Baird 2002): (1) to help families cope with and manage the continuing stresses inherent in chronic disease management, as a team, rather than as individuals; (2) to mobilize the patient's natural support system to enhance family closeness, increase mutually supportive interactions among family members, and build additional extra familial support, thus improving disease management and the health and well-being of the patient and other family members; and (3) to minimize intrafamilial hostility and criticism and to reduce the adverse effects of external stress and disease-related trauma on family life.

More specifically, according to Weihs and colleagues, family-focused interventions should

1. help family members agree on and collaborate on a program of disease management in ways that are consistent with their beliefs and operational style;
2. help family members manage stress by preventing the disease from dominating family life and sacrificing normal developmental and personal goals;
3. help the family deal with the losses that chronic illness can create;
4. mobilize the family's natural support system to provide education and support for all family members involved in disease management;
5. reduce the social isolation and resulting anxiety and depression that disease management can create in both the patient and other family members; and
6. reorganize the family, with adjustments of roles and expectations as needed, to ensure optimal patient self-care. (2002, p. 25)

These goals shift care from a patient focus to a broader systems perspective, which considers the relational context of the family as the target for intervention. As seen in the above studies, this shift improves the health and well-being of patients and families struggling with the management of chronic disease. Many of these principles can apply equally to chronic psychiatric illnesses.

PSYCHIATRY

This section reviews the studies of family interventions in psychiatry that are most pertinent for the inpatient psychiatrist. The first family intervention studies were of families of patients with schizophrenia. Over time, their application in many other illnesses has also been studied. The American Psychiatric Association (APA) includes family interventions in many of their Practice Guidelines; the guidelines pertinent for the inpatient psychiatrist are reviewed in each section below.

Schizophrenia

Families have become the main caregivers for patients with schizophrenia, because of the reduction in length of hospitalization owing to managed care and the lack of funding for community psychiatric programs. It is not uncommon for family care providers to feel overwhelmed and confused; many family caregivers lack an understanding of the illness and have inadequate skills to manage aberrant behavior. To address this need for education, investigators developed family-based psychosocial interventions for patients with schizophrenia and their family health care providers. These interventions focus primarily on providing education about the illness and improving coping skills (Anderson, Hogarty, and Reiss 1980). Family psychoeducation for schizophrenia is based on the premise that the patient has a brain disorder and that families need to be supported in their care of the mentally ill person. The emphasis on the biological aspect of the illness is intended to correct the misperception that families somehow cause the illness. This unfortunate misperception originated in early work with patients with schizophrenia and their families. Kasanin, Knight, and Sage (1934) were among the first to implicate parenting problems in schizophrenia, singling out maternal rejection or overprotection. Fromm-Reichman

(1948, p. 265) stated, "[T]he schizophrenic is painfully distrustful and resentful of other people due to the severe early warp and rejection he encountered in important people in his infancy and childhood, as a rule mainly the schizophrenogenic mother." Uncontrolled studies developed concepts such as marital schism and marital skew to explain schizophrenia in the child (Lidz et al. 1957). Family systems theorists continued the preoccupation with the dysfunctional family, developing other concepts such as the "double bind" theory of schizophrenia (Bateson et al. 1956), which involved disordered communications within the family unit, the mother being the most disordered family member. Jackson (1957, p. 184) wrote that "perhaps the next phase will include a study of schizophrenia as a family-borne disease involving a complicated host-vector-recipient cycle that includes much more than can be connoted by the term, schizophrenogenic mother. One could even speculate whether schizophrenia as it is known today would exist if parthenogenesis were the usual mode of propagation of the human species, or if women were impersonally impregnated and gave birth to infants who were reared by state nurses in a communal setting." Not surprisingly, these comments have caused tremendous anguish for family members and a deep distrust of psychiatry. Families of persons with schizophrenia have therefore kept away from a profession that has blamed them rather than embraced them. Thus, there is a purposeful emphasis on the biological etiology of schizophrenia in the psychoeducational programs.

The psychoeducational programs are also based on the premise that healthy coping strategies for families can be taught. The most frequent types of components in psychoeducational programs are training in problem-solving skills, the development of positive communication, and increased social involvement for the family. Family psychoeducation includes the provision of emotional support, education about the illness, and highlighting resources during periods of crisis. Emphasis is placed on families learning from each other, as mutual support is considered to be one of the main therapeutic factors in these programs. The key components of psychoeducational treatment for schizophrenia were identified in 1999 by the World Schizophrenia Fellowship. Clear principles for psychoeducation were laid out; they included optimizing medication management and addressing the family's feelings of loss. Table 4.1 outlines the essential elements of the psychoeducational approach for schizophrenia.

TABLE 4.1
Essential Elements of Psychoeducation:
Principles for Working with Families

Coordinate all elements of treatment to ensure that everyone is working toward the
  same goals in a collaborative relationship.
Pay attention to the patient's social as well as clinical needs.
Provide optimal medication management.
Listen to families and treat them as equal partners.
Explore family members' expectations of the treatment program and for the patient.
Assess the family's strengths and limitations in their ability to support the patient.
Help resolve conflict through sensitive response to emotional distress.
Address feelings of loss.
Provide relevant information to the family and patient at appropriate times.
Provide an explicit crisis plan and professional response.
Help improve communication among family members.
Provide training for the family in structured problem-solving techniques.
Encourage the family to expand their social support networks.
Be flexible in meeting the needs of families.
Provide the family with easy access to a professional in case of need.

Source: McFarlane et al. 2003. Reprinted with permission.

A large number of controlled clinical trials support the use of family
psychoeducation in the treatment of schizophrenia. The Schizophrenia
Patients Outcome Research Team project and the APA Practice Guidelines for Schizophrenia include specific recommendations about family
psychoeducation. The provision of family psychoeducation has been
found to reduce the relapse rate for patients to 15 percent per year compared to 30–40 percent for patients who do not receive this intervention.
Most recommendations call for multifamily group treatment, but there is
a subgroup of families that does well with single-family psychoeducation.
This subgroup consists of families with low expressed emotion and whose
ill family member has a good response to medication (McFarlane and
Deakins 2002).

Despite the clear benefit to patients and families, very few psychoeducational programs are available. Therefore, families themselves have developed
community-based education programs. These programs differ from the pro-
fessionally led psychoeducational programs in that they are run by family
member volunteers. These groups are focused on helping the family mem-

bers rather than on altering the behavior or attending to the needs of the ill individuals. This type of group is discussed in more detail in Chapter 11.

Cultural and ethnic differences in family-based treatment outcomes have been found but are sparsely researched. In Mexican immigrant families who received behavioral family therapy, the ill family member actually relapsed at a higher rate than did comparable patients who received traditional case management (Telles et al. 1995). In Spain, no difference in patient relapse rate was found between patients whose families participated in psychoeducational programs compared to those whose families were in the control group (Canive et al. 1996). It is unclear what these findings mean, but cultural differences do need to be taken into account when creating family interventions.

Bipolar Disorder

It is well recognized that medication alone is not sufficient treatment for bipolar disorder and that psychosocial treatment is needed if relapse rates are to improve (Miklowitz et al. 2003). At a National Institute of Mental Health conference in 1989, adjunct psychosocial therapy was declared the most underdeveloped area in the treatment of bipolar disorder. Despite the research that has been done since that time, what type of psychosocial intervention is optimal remains unclear. In general nonspecific ways, families can contribute positively to patient outcome by: assisting with treatment (such as compliance with medication), monitoring the illness, noticing side effects, adhering to scheduled appointments, and promoting good health-maintenance strategies (such as adequate exercise, sleep hygiene, and maintaining a balanced diet) (Clarkin et al. 1998; Keitner and Miller 1990; Keitner et al. 1995; Ryan et al. 2005). Patient outcome is also improved by helping the patients and their families with training in problem-solving skills and communication (Miklowitz et al. 2003; Miklowitz and Goldstein 1997).

Patients who received family-focused therapy had fewer relapses (35%) and longer survival intervals (periods without relapse) (73.5 weeks) than patients who received crisis management (54%; 53.2 weeks) (Miklowitz and Goldstein 1997). Family-focused therapy consisted of 21 sessions of psychoeducation, training in communication, and training in problem-solving skills over nine months. Crisis management consisted of two sessions of family education plus sessions on crisis intervention as needed. Patients who received family-focused therapy also showed reductions in mood symptoms and better adherence to medication, both of which were sustained at the two-year follow-up. Rea and colleagues (2003) improved on this study by controlling for the number of therapist contact hours and found relapse rates with family-focused therapy of 28 percent compared with 60 percent in the crisis management group. The rate of rehospitalization in the group with family-focused therapy was also lower (12% versus 60%). In an attempt to further increase the response to treatment, Miklowitz and colleagues (2003) developed an approach that combined individual therapy and family intervention as an adjunctive treatment for bipolar disorder. This integrated family and individual therapy consisted of a maximum of 25 sessions each of family-focused therapy and individual therapy consisting of interpersonal and social rhythm therapy, in alternating weeks, over the course of one year. Interpersonal and social rhythm therapy focuses on interpersonal problems, identifying triggers for social rhythm disruptions, stabilization of daily routines, and prevention of relapse. Patients who receive integrated family and individual therapy had significantly longer survival intervals than those receiving case management (42.5 versus 34.5 weeks). Both treatment groups showed improvement in symptoms, but patients in the group with integrated family and individual therapy showed greater reduction in depressive symptoms over one year than those in the group receiving only crisis management. This study yielded some additional interesting facts. For example, depressive symptoms appear to be more amenable to integrated family and individual therapy than do manic symptoms, and, despite many therapeutic sessions being available to patients and their families, most patients and families did not use all the available sessions.

What about expressed emotion ratings in bipolar patients and their families? In the Miklowitz Colorado Treatment/Outcome Project and the integrated family and individual therapy study described above, patients with high EE relatives did not relapse at higher rates over the two-year follow-up nor did they relapse sooner than patients from families with low EE relatives (Kimand and Miklowitz 2004). However, when the severity of the patients' symptoms rather than relapse status was assessed, patients from high EE families had significantly higher levels of depression throughout than did patients from low EE families, regardless of the treatment condition. The greater severity of depressive symptoms may be more pertinent to issues of disability, functional impairment, and quality-of-life than the frequency or timing of relapses. It is worthwhile to emphasize the importance of these findings as they relate to depressive symptoms. Patients with bipolar disorder and their families indicate that the depressive phase of the illness causes more difficulty, more disability and functional impairment, and poorer quality of life than does the manic phase (Calabrese et al. 2004). Thus, interventions that specifically target the depressive phase of the illness must continue to be developed.

The interventions described above assess only patient outcome. What about interventions that assess family outcome? We know that families cope better when they understand that their relative's problematic behavior is caused by illness, not "bad behavior" (Perlick et al. 1999). The provision of multifamily group therapy can significantly improve family functioning. In a well-designed study, 92 patients with bipolar disorder were randomly assigned to three treatment types: pharmacotherapy alone, pharmacotherapy and individual therapy, and pharmacotherapy and multifamily psychoeducation group intervention (Keitner, Ryan, et al. 2003). The multifamily group treatment consisted of four to six families (and the patients) who met for six sessions with co-therapists. Although the number of subjects in each treatment group who recovered from their episode did not differ significantly nor did the time to recovery differ among the three groups, the provision of multifamily group therapy significantly improved family functioning.

In summary, for persons with bipolar disorder, adjunctive psychoeducational and/or psychotherapeutic approaches improve the efficacy of treatment over pharmacotherapy alone, especially in delaying the emergence of new episodes. These psychosocial interventions are considered to be an important part of the long-term management of bipolar disorder (Vieta and Colom 2004). The development of interventions that target the depressive phase of the illness is of primary importance.

Major Depression

Patients with major depression show greater improvement and significant reductions in depression and suicidal ideation when treatment includes a family therapy component than when it does not. Miller and colleagues (2005) studied 105 patients with major depression discharged from the inpatient unit, and their families. Patients were randomly assigned to one of four treatment groups: (1) pharmacotherapy alone, (2) combined pharmacotherapy and cognitive therapy, (3) combined pharmacotherapy and family therapy, and (4) combined pharmacotherapy and cognitive therapy and family therapy. Patients with poor family functioning who were assigned to receive family therapy were described as "matched" (the treatment matched the need), and patients with poor family functioning who were assigned to cognitive therapy were described as "mismatched." The study showed that patients who received matched treatment had significantly greater improvement than patients who received mismatched treatment. Treatment continued for 24 weeks. The family therapy component was conducted using the Problem-Centered Systems Therapy of the Family (Epstein et al. 2003; Ryan et al. 2005), which is a systems-oriented brief therapy composed of four major stages (assessment, contracting, treatment, and closure) and emphasizes problem solving. Table 4.2 outlines the principles and the macro stages of this therapy.

For outpatients with mild to moderate major depression, couples therapy has been found to be as efficacious as, and preferable to, antidepressant medication (Leff et al. 2000). Leff and colleagues studied 77 outpatients and their partners who were randomized to either antidepressant medication or couples therapy and were followed for one year. Desipramine was the initial medication, and an SSRI was substituted if a patient experienced side effects or did not respond to the medication. The couples therapy consisted of interventions such as interruption of problematic behavioral transactions and setting of tasks. The protocol allowed for 12 to 20 sessions.

In summary, family treatment delivered using stringently controlled manuals is efficacious for depressive illnesses. For inpatients with major depression, family treatment after discharge is recommended.

Obsessive-Compulsive Disorder

For obsessive-compulsive disorder (OCD), family treatment produces a superior outcome to individual therapy. Patients whose family members participate in family group treatment have a greater reduction in OCD symptoms and an improved mood compared to patients whose relatives do not participate. In one small study of 28 treatment-refractory patients with OCD (Grunes, Neziroglu, and McKay 2001), the families randomized to family group treatment participated in an 8-week psychoeducational group designed to reduce accommodation to OCD symptoms. A reduction in OCD symptoms also occurs with family group treatment that provides edu-

TABLE 4.2
Family Therapy Using Problem-Centered Systems Therapy of the Family

Ten Principles

1. Emphasis on "macro" stages of treatment
2. Establishment of a collaborative set between therapist and family members
3. Open, direct communication with the family
4. Focus on the family's responsibility for change
5. Emphasis on current problems
6. Focus on behavioral change
7. Emphasis on assessment
8. Focus on family strengths
9. Inclusion of the entire family
10. A time-limited nature

Stages of Treatment

The *assessment stage* is the most important. It is the stage in which the therapist orients the family to the treatment process and establishes an open, collaborative relationship with the family. The therapist and the family identify current problems, including the presenting problem and problems within the six dimensions—roles, communication, affective involvement, affective responsiveness, behavior control, and problem solving. At the end of the assessment, the therapist formulates hypotheses regarding the factors and/or processes that appear to be causally associated with the family's identified problems. The therapist and the family together clarify and agree on a list of problems, which then becomes the foundation for treatment.

In the *contracting stage*, the goal is for the therapist and family to prepare a contract that delineates mutual expectations, goals, and commitments regarding therapy. Problems are prioritized according to their importance to the family. The therapist may have to pre-empt this priority list if issues of safety are involved and the family does not identify risk situations as problematic.

In the *treatment stage*, the therapist and family members implement strategies and negotiate ways to change the identified behaviors that contribute to the problems. The goal is to produce behavioral change in the family by setting and monitoring tasks that the family will work on between sessions.

In the *closure stage*, the therapist reviews the course of treatment with the family, and long-term goals as well as optional follow-up visits are discussed.

Source: Adapted from Epstein and Bishop 1981, Epstein et al. 2003, and Ryan et al. 2005.

cation about the illness, teaching about family contracting for behavior change, and practicing direct exposure (Van Noppen et al. 1997). Group family therapy has been favorably compared to individual family therapy in children and adolescents (Barrett, Healy-Farrell, and March 2004). Group family treatment uses a cognitive-behavioral protocol with parental and sibling components. The family component focuses on managing the child's OCD and teaching parents and siblings strategies to manage their own distress within the context of the OCD. Follow-up consists of two booster sessions (1 month and 3 months after treatment), each running for approximately 1.5 hours. Parental sessions focus on psychoeducation, problem-solving skills, and strategies to reduce parental involvement in the child's symptoms, along with encouraging family support of home-based exposure and response-prevention trials. The program emphasizes that coping strategies need to be practiced as a family on a daily basis. This protocol is an example of a well-designed psychoeducational program that can be implemented in conjunction with the treatment of the individual child or adolescent. Table 4.3 outlines details of the interventions provided in this study.

Family intervention for OCD can be started on an inpatient unit. Family involvement in rituals can be reduced by training family members to monitor the patient's behavior and to encourage patient self-exposure in a noncritical manner (Thornicroft, Colson, and Marks 1991). With this family-based intervention, severely ill inpatients with OCD had a reduction in symptoms of 60 percent at the six-month follow-up. In summary, OCD is particularly amenable to family-based behavioral interventions because of the ability to define clear behavioral goals in treatment.

Borderline Personality Disorder

The inclusion of family members in the treatment of persons with borderline personality disorder is controversial. It had always been assumed that the families of persons with borderline personality disorder were "over-involved, separation-resistant," and that the mothers were "dependency generating"; but when these families were studied, they were found to be more likely to be underinvolved (Gunderson, Berkowitz, and Ruiz-Sancho 1997, p. 448). These families tended to be ostracized by both patients and therapists; some therapists would warn their patients to stay away from their families. Sometimes, at a therapist's encouragement, the family was brought in to listen to the complaints of mistreatment from the patient. Gunderson states that while he erroneously contributed to this literature of vilification of the families in the past, he now actively supports the involvement of families as important allies in the treatment of patients with borderline personality disorder. Gunderson's McLean psychoeducational program reflects a dramatic shift in practice for the management of borderline personality disorder. Borderline personality disorder had been treated with individual

TABLE 4.3
Cognitive Family Behavioral Treatment for OCD

Session No.	Child Session	[Joint Session]	Parent/Sibling Session
1.		• Psychoeducation • Developing a neurobehavioral framework • Forming an expert team • Externalizing OCD	
2.	• Introducing tool kit • Mapping OCD		• Psychoeducation continued
3.	• More mapping • Understanding anxiety and body clues • Relaxation games		• Physiology of anxiety • Parental anxiety management
4.	• Introduction to thoughts and feelings • Self-talk and bossing back OCD		• Psychoeducation of OCD • How OCD affects siblings • Anxiety management for siblings
5.	• Thought traps of OCD • Probability and responsibility • Responses to OCD thoughts		• Cognitive biases of OCD • Rational responses to OCD • Appropriate ways of responding to OCD demands
6.	• Step plans • Goal setting • Introduce E/RP steps		• Introduction to E/RP • Developing a fear hierarchy
7.	• Mapping OCD • Review E/RP steps • Rewards for partial successes		• Managing behavioral difficulties • More mapping OCD • Fear hierarchies
8.	• Mapping OCD • Review E/RP steps • Mapping parental and sibling involvement and accommodation		• Mapping parental and sibling involvement and accommodation
9.		• Family problem-solving strategies • The 6-step plan • Negotiating disengagement of parental and sibling accommodation and involvement	
10.	• Mapping OCD • Review E/RP steps • Develop step plans for new activities to replace OCD		• Who is your child without OCD? • Activities to introduce into child's life to replace OCD
11.	• Mapping OCD • Review E/RP steps/ new activities steps • Mapping support networks		• Overcoming obstacles in withdrawal of accommodation • Supports networks

(continued)

TABLE 4.3
Cognitive Family Behavioral Treatment for OCD (continued)

Session No.	Child Session	[Joint Session]	Parent/Sibling Session

12.	• Mapping OCD
	• Review E/RP steps/
	  new activities steps
	• OCD in disguise: doubt,
	  slowness, avoidance
			• Reviewing sibling accom-
			  modation
			• Identifying disguises of OCD
			  and ways of managing them

13.	• Review E/RP steps/
	  new activities steps
	• Mapping what OCD might look
	  like in the future
			• Planning futures without OCD

14.		• Reviewing tool kit • Reward ceremonies	
15.	• Booster 1 (1 month) • Review tool kit and prepare step plans		• Parental support • Sibling support
16.	• Booster 2 (3 months) • Review tool kit and prepare step plans		• Parental support • Sibling support

Source: Adapted from Barrett, Healy-Farrell, and March 2004.
Notes: Sessions 4, 8, 12, 15, and 16 were sibling sessions. Sibling session 1 occurred with siblings alone, session 2 with siblings and parents, and for session 3 siblings were with OCD child. This sometimes varied to suit the individual families or the group members.
    OCD = obsessive-compulsive disorder; E/RP = exposure and response prevention.

psychotherapy, most recently dialectical behavior therapy, a variant of cognitive behavioral therapy (Linehan et al. 1991). Now, family therapy is recommended as an adjunctive treatment for this disorder. Gunderson's study of families of patients with this condition identifies difficulties with communication, conflict, and anger as major problems, as well as struggling with how to manage the patient's suicidality (Gunderson and Lyoo 1997).

In Gunderson's family treatment program, borderline personality disorder is conceptualized as a disorder that is caused by the interplay of many factors, and the patients are portrayed as both disabled and willful. Family history is not discussed and families are told that there is not enough information available to give a meaningful answer to questions about etiology. Families and patients are encouraged to look toward the future and to learn new coping strategies. The first phase of their treatment consists of one to four "joining" sessions. Each family is met with individually, listened to, and given educational material about the diagnosis, course, and treatment of borderline personality disorder. This session is followed by a half-day workshop attended by up to 30 family members of patients. The previously distributed material is reviewed in detail, then there is a question-and-answer period. The general atmosphere is designed to be informal, encouraging a sense of group cohesion. The expectation is that people will benefit from exposure to others dealing with similar experiences. Guidelines are presented to the families and the format for the next phase is explained. The next phase consists of multifamily group treatment. Each family is encouraged to present a problem and the other participants are asked to help solve the problem. In this phase, the families are encouraged to be less crisis oriented, to maintain stable family patterns, and to develop predictable times of contact with the patient that are not tied to threats or rages or other crisis. Family members are encouraged to listen to the patient's attacks without becoming angry and defensive and, if a tirade is prolonged, to leave and not tolerate abuse; outbursts can be discussed with the patient at a later time, when the patient is calm. In these sessions, family members can express the extent of discomfort they experience during such angry outbursts. A key intervention is to encourage the family to present a united front to the patient. These multifamily groups meet for 1.5 hours every other week. In the McLean program, families usually participate in these meeting for about 18 months. The results of the family treatment include increased communication and decreased family conflict. Table 4.4 outlines the principles of the McLean family intervention program.

Alcohol Abuse and Dependence

Family treatment encourages positive changes by motivating alcoholic persons to enter treatment and, additionally, results in improved coping skills for family members. Thirty-eight controlled studies of marital and family therapy support the use of family treatment in alcohol dependence (O'Farrell and Fals-Stewart 2003). One type of family therapy, behavioral couples therapy, is more effective than individual treatment at increasing abstinence and also improves relationship functioning, reduces social costs incurred as a result of alcoholism, reduces the incidence of domestic violence, and limits emotional problems in the children of participants (O'Farrell et al. 2003). The behavioral couples therapy program is intensive and requires a time

TABLE 4.4
*Guidelines for Families with Relatives
with Borderline Personality Disorder*

Recovery takes time. Go slow. Crises do resolve.

Keep things cool. Enthusiasm and disagreements are normal. Tone them down.

Don't ignore threats of self-destructiveness. Express concern. Discuss with professionals.

Maintain family routines as much as possible. Don't forsake good times. Don't withdraw from friends.

Listen. Don't get defensive in the face of criticisms. However unfair, say little. Allow yourself to be hurt.

Source: Adapted from Gunderson, Berkowitz, and Ruiz-Sancho 1997.

commitment of up to 22 sessions over six months. There are 10 to 12 weekly pregroup sessions with each couple, followed by 10 two-hour multifamily groups. Behavioral couples therapy implements a daily sobriety contract that includes administration of Antabuse under spousal supervision.

For patients with alcohol dependence who are discharged from the inpatient unit, family treatment can therefore be confidently recommended. Table 4.5 outlines the essential elements of behavioral couples therapy (O'Farrell and Fals-Stewart 2000).

Anorexia Nervosa

Adolescents with anorexia nervosa benefit from family therapy, especially when the parents take an active role with the adolescent (Asen 2002). Single-family therapy and multifamily psychoeducational groups are equally effective in restoring weight (Geist et al. 2000). For adults with anorexia nervosa, family therapy is comparable to individual psychotherapy and both produce superior results than treatment without either (Dare et al. 2001).

PRACTICE GUIDELINES

The American Psychiatric Association (APA) recognizes the validity of family-based interventions in their Practice Guidelines. Guidelines for each disease addressed discuss the etiology of the illness and outline the current evidence-based treatments. The second edition of the Guidelines for Schizophrenia (APA, Work Group on Schizophrenia 2004) outlines in detail the

TABLE 4.5
Behavioral Couples Therapy (BCT) for the Treatment of Alcoholism

A. Sobriety contract
1. A daily sobriety contract, in which the patient states intention not to drink or use drugs that day (in the tradition of one day at a time) and the spouse expresses support for the patient's efforts to stay abstinent.
2. For alcoholic patients who are medically cleared and willing, daily Antabuse ingestion witnessed and verbally reinforced by the spouse also is part of the sobriety contract.
3. The spouse records the performance of the daily contract on a calendar provided by the therapist.
4. Both partners agree not to discuss past drinking or fears about future drinking at home to prevent substance-related conflicts, which can trigger relapse. Reserve these discussions for the therapy sessions.
5. At the start of each couple session, the therapist reviews the sobriety contract calendar to see how well each spouse has done his or her part. If the sobriety contract includes 12-step meetings or urine drug screens, these are also marked on the calendar and reviewed. The calendar provides an ongoing record of progress that is rewarded verbally at each session. The couple performs the behaviors of the sobriety contract in each session to highlight its importance and to let the therapist observe how the couple carries out the contract.

B. Provision of behavioral assignments to increase positive feelings, shared activities, and constructive communication
1. Catch your partner doing something nice: each spouse notices and acknowledges one pleasing behavior performed by the partner each day.
2. Caring day assignment: each person plans ahead to surprise the spouse with a day when they do some special things to show their caring.
3. Share rewarding activities: each activity must involve both spouses, either with their children or other adults or not, and it can be at or away from home.
4. Teach communication skills.

C. Relapse prevention
At the end of weekly BCT sessions, each couple completes a continuing recovery plan, which is reviewed at quarterly follow-up visits for an additional two years.

Source: Adapted from O'Farrell and Fals-Stewart 2000.

importance of involving the family in the management of the illness, recommending that the psychiatrist establish a therapeutic alliance with the family and address the family's needs, especially during an acute episode. The Guidelines for Schizophrenia recommend routinely meeting with family members to obtain information and to provide information on the management of the illness. They state, "Educational meetings and survival workshops that teach families how to cope with schizophrenia and referrals to local chapters of patient and family organizations such as the National Alliance for the Mentally Ill (NAMI) may be helpful and are recommended. Families may be under considerable stress, particularly if the patient has been exhibiting dangerous or unstable behavior" (p. 5). The stable phase, the guidelines recommend, should be used to educate the family about signs of relapse and advise them on developing a plan of action in case these signs appear. They also state that family members receive support, training in problem solving, and training in communication. The role of family members in helping patients comply with their medication is emphasized. The availability of manuals, workbooks, and videotapes for family members is pointed out. The guidelines indicate that the Substance Abuse and Mental Health Services Administration (SAMHSA) is developing resource kits on family interventions in schizophrenia. The efficacy of family interventions in preventing relapse and improving patient functioning and family well-being is emphasized. Specifically, the guidelines state, "On the basis of the evidence, persons with schizophrenia and their families who have ongoing contact with each other should be offered a family intervention, the key elements of which include a duration of at least 9 months, illness education, crisis intervention, emotional support and training in how to cope with illness symptoms and related problems" (p. 21). The Practice Guidelines for Bipolar Disorder (APA, Work Group on Bipolar Disorder 2002) and for Major Depression (APA 2000) also recommend early family involvement and present the known findings about the efficacy of family-based interventions. Practice guidelines for other disorders, such as panic disorder, eating disorders, and substance abuse disorders, similarly recommend early involvement of the family and provide evidence of the efficacy of marital or family therapy as a psychosocial intervention.

SUMMARY

Family-based interventions are a significant contribution to psychiatric practice. Many randomized clinical trials have demonstrated that family-based interventions reduce relapse rates, improve patients' recovery, and improve family well-being among participants (McFarlane et al. 2003). The psychiatrist can therefore confidently commend family interventions to patients and their families, backing up this advice with relevant treatment studies.

PART THREE

Mastering Skills

CHAPTER FIVE

Abbreviated Assessment of the Family

This chapter describes how to complete an abbreviated family assessment of an inpatient and the patient's family. The authors teach the McMaster assessment model and the Problem-Centered Systems Therapy of the Family (Epstein and Bishop 1981) and utilize this model in outpatient work with families and in training of residents in the outpatient department. For work with inpatients and their families, we use an abbreviated assessment, because of the time constraints of inpatient work. We have extracted key elements of the McMaster assessment process: the development of a problem list, a three-question inquiry for each of the identified problems, and pertinent questions drawn as needed from the different dimensions of family functioning. Using an abbreviated assessment helps structure inpatient family meetings. Because time is limited, the inpatient meeting must accomplish additional goals, such as psychoeducation and discharge planning. Residents who work on the inpatient units are at the beginning of their training and have not yet learned how to fully assess a family. These key elements are sufficient for structuring a time-limited inpatient family meeting. Two case examples illustrate the use of two structured assessment tools: the McMaster Model of Family Functioning and the Global Assessment of Relational Functioning.

An inpatient family meeting serves multiple purposes, such as to provide information about the patient's illness, to offer support to the family, and to provide psychoeducation. Including the family in the patient's treatment enhances the clinical care of the patient. We have borrowed aspects from the Global Assessment of Relational Functioning (APA 2000) and the McMaster Model of Family Functioning (Epstein et al. 2003) to create practical and useful tools for assessing the family in a short time. For example, by constructing a list of problems and taking a brief history of each problem, the resident can gather some basic data without becoming bogged down in too much detail. Before meeting the family, the resident and treatment team should assemble all pertinent information about the patient, such as precipitants of hospitalization, known family concerns, medical issues, and the patient's course of illness. This information is compiled from the initial assessment at the time of admission to the hospital, the inpatient interdisciplinary assessment, and collateral information from outpatient health care providers and the family. Having an understanding of all of the assessment material helps the resident become familiar with the pertinent problem areas before meeting with the family. Of course, the resident should be aware that other concerns, especially intimacy issues, may not have been identified in the assessments, and he or she should be aware that these concerns may emerge.

ASSESSMENT OF THE FAMILY

A family assessment, full or abbreviated, is a "blueprint" of the family's problems, strengths, and weaknesses. Think of a family assessment as being similar to a mental status examination. The assessment gives the family the opportunity to identify and explore problems, strengths, weaknesses, and patterns of interaction.

The initial stages of therapy are known to have significant clinical impact, and an assessment, of either the individual or the family, is usually considered the first stage of therapy (Budman and Gurman 1988). Families can gain a greater understanding of their problems during an assessment and make changes immediately based on this new understanding. For example, when the son expresses a desire to spend more time with his father, the opportunity exists for that to happen immediately if the father is receptive. Generally, after the family assessment, there is a "window of opportunity" when the family can be most actively engaged. While the patient is in the hospital, families willingly participate in family meetings, and resolution of simple family problems can often be accomplished at that time. After the initial sessions, however, reluctance to engage with problems sets in and other life responsibilities return to the foreground for the family, thus reducing their willingness to attend additional meetings. Consequently, it is important to "strike while the iron is hot," when the patient is still hospitalized and the family is highly motivated to attend meetings.

During a family assessment, faulty notions regarding the cause and management of the illness can be replaced with models that provide for optimal functioning for all family members. Patients and families are inclined to create explanatory models of their experience of illness and to formulate hypotheses regarding the cause of the illness. Such patient- and family-constructed explanatory models of illness, if left unchecked, may create barriers to clinical progress. For example, the patient who believes that hypertension is the consequence of "being tense" will take antihypertensive medicine only when feeling anxious (Kleinman 1988). For families who are able to meet several times, the opportunity exists to complete a full assessment, rather than an abbreviated assessment.

How Does Assessment Differ from Treatment?

A family assessment, full or abbreviated, provides an understanding of the family's overall functioning. An abbreviated assessment can be completed when time is limited. After the family assessment, the resident may recommend family treatment. The family decides if they want to enter treatment. In treatment, the family actively negotiates to resolve problems identified in the assessment.

What Can Be Accomplished in an Abbreviated Assessment?

The resident establishes and maintains an alliance with the family by engaging each family member in the assessment process. Always listening carefully and feeding back each family member's perspective on each of the identified problems ensures that each family member feels heard and understood. The family is successfully engaged when family members say to themselves, "This doctor understands my perspective. This doctor gets it. I think I can work with this doctor." Of course, the physician must be scrupulously fair and avoid taking sides when working to form an alliance with the family. Family members are more likely to listen to others, negotiate, and compromise when each person feels heard and understood.

Raising the consciousness of the family is the first step toward behavioral change. In the course of the assessment, each member tells his or her side of the problems and has the experience of being listened to by the other family members; from this a fuller understanding of the problems unfolds. The family that comes together and discusses their issues, perhaps for the first time with a neutral third party, has taken an important step in moving toward problem resolution. When the family has identified and described all problems, the physician reviews the list of problems with the family and secures their agreement that the list reflects an accurate summary of their issues. Where family members disagree on a problem, they can "agree to disagree."

When Does the Treatment Begin?

If the family wants to enter into family treatment, the resident makes an outpatient referral and, with the family's written permission, forwards a summary of the family assessment to the outpatient practitioner. Family treatment is beyond the scope of most hospitalizations and is usually completed on an outpatient basis. Sometimes, however, the family will request to continue working with the inpatient physician in family treatment, and several family meetings can be held before discharge. The family that is ready for family treatment (1) has completed a family assessment, (2) is aware of each member's perspective on all of the issues, and (3) has agreed to actively work to make changes.

What Is the Responsibility of the Resident?

In the abbreviated family assessment, the resident is responsible for identifying family factors, in order to construct a biopsychosocial case formulation and treatment plan. It is important that, after identifying these factors, the resident consider whether a full family assessment is indicated. In some cases, the resident may have the time and expertise to provide this service on the inpatient unit. More commonly, the resident will refer the family to an outpatient family therapist.

What Is the Responsibility of the Family?

In the abbreviated family assessment, the family is responsible for participating in the inpatient meeting. Frequently, some family members do not attend the inpatient family meeting, for reasons such as school attendance or work schedule. A *full* family assessment, however, requires the attendance of all pertinent family members. During assessment, the family's responsibility is to provide open and honest accounts of the family's problems and functioning. Their responsibility during family *treatment* is to actively work on problem resolution.

STRUCTURED ASSESSMENT TOOLS

The Global Assessment of Relational Functioning

The Global Assessment of Relational Functioning (GARF) (GAP 1996) is a composite of the three most researched family assessment tools: the Beavers Systems Model (Beavers and Hampson 1990), the Olsen Circumplex Model (Olsen 1996), and the McMaster Model (Epstein et al. 2003). The GARF provides a numerical score of the family's functioning and is used much like the Global Assessment of Functioning (GAF) for individuals. The GARF is found in Appendix B of the DSM IV-TR (APA 2000). It assesses three areas—interactional problem solving, organization, and emotional climate—on a scale of 1 to 99 as follows:

1–20 Family is too dysfunctional to retain continuity, contact, and attachment.

21–40 Family is obviously and seriously dysfunctional.

41–60 Family has occasional times of satisfactory functioning but unsatisfactory relationships predominate.

61–80 Family functioning is somewhat unsatisfactory.

81–100 Family functioning is satisfactory.

Table 5.1 gives a fuller description of the rating scales. When applied in detail, the GARF provides an understanding of the overall functioning of the family. It is completed after the family assessment meeting. An extensive description of its use is given by Yingling et al. (1998).

The McMaster Model of Family Functioning

The McMaster Model of Family Functioning (MMFF) is the assessment tool that is used most commonly throughout this book. The MMFF has specific questions pertaining to six dimensions of family functioning: roles, problem solving, communication, affective responsiveness, affective involvement,

TABLE 5.1
GARF Levels of Family Functioning

Interactional Problem Solving	Organization	Emotional Climate
(Skills in negotiating goals, rules, and routines; adaptability to stress; communication skills; ability to resolve conflict)	(Maintenance of interpersonal roles and subsystem boundaries; hierarchical functioning; coalitions and distribution of power, control, and responsibility)	(Tone and range of feelings; quality of caring, empathy, and attachment/commitment; sharing of values; mutual affective responsiveness, respect, and regard; quality of sexual functioning)
81–100: Agreed-on patterns or routines exist that help meet the usual needs of each family/ couple member; there is flexibility for change in response to unusual demands or events; and occasional conflicts and stressful transitions are resolved through problem solving, communication, and negotiation.	81–100: There is a shared understanding and agreement about roles and appropriate tasks; decision making is established for each functional area; and there is recognition of the unique characteristics and merit of each subsystem (e.g., parents/ spouses, siblings, and individuals).	81–100: There is a situationally appropriate, optimistic atmosphere in the family; a wide range of feelings is freely expressed and managed within the family; and there is a general atmosphere of warmth, caring, and sharing of values among all family members. Sexual relations of adult members are satisfactory.
61–80: Daily routines are present but there is some pain and difficulty in responding to the unusual. Some conflicts remain unresolved but do not disrupt family functioning.	61–80: Decision making is usually competent, but efforts at control of one another often are greater than necessary or are ineffective. Individuals and relationships are clearly demarcated, but sometimes a specific subsystem is depreciated or scapegoated.	61–80: A range of feeling is expressed, but instances of emotional blocking or tension are evident. Warmth and caring are present but are marred by a family member's irritability and frustrations. Sexual activity of adult members may be reduced or problematic
41–60: Communication is frequently inhibited by unresolved conflicts that interfere with daily routines; there is significant difficulty in adapting to family stress and transitional change.	41–60: Decision making is competent and effective only intermittently; either excessive rigidity or significant lack of structure is evident at these times; individual needs are quite often submerged by a partner or coalition.	41–60: Pain or ineffective anger or emotional deadness interfere with family enjoyment; although there is some warmth and support for members, it is usually unequally distributed. Troublesome sexual difficulties between adults are often present.

(continued)

TABLE 5.1
GARF Levels of Family Functioning (continued)

Interactional Problem Solving	Organization	Emotional Climate
(Skills in negotiating goals, rules, and routines; adaptability to stress; communication skills; ability to resolve conflict)	(Maintenance of interpersonal roles and subsystem boundaries; hierarchical functioning; coalitions and distribution of power, control, and responsibility)	(Tone and range of feelings; quality of caring, empathy, and attachment/commitment; sharing of values; mutual affective responsiveness, respect, and regard; quality of sexual functioning)
21–40: Family/couple routines do not meet the needs of members; they are grimly adhered to or blithely ignored; life cycle changes, such as departures from or entries into the relational unit, generate painful conflict and obviously frustrating failures of problem solving.	21–40: Decision making is tyrannical or quite ineffective. The unique characteristics of individuals are unappreciated or ignored by either rigid or confusingly fluid coalitions.	21–40: There are infrequent periods of enjoyment of life together; frequent distancing or open hostility reflects significant conflicts that remain unresolved and quite painful. Sexual dysfunction among adult members is commonplace.
1–20: Family/couple routines are negligible (e.g., no mealtime, sleeping, or waking schedule); family members often do not know where others are or when they will be in or out; there is little effective communciation among family members.	1–20: Family/couple members are not organized in such a way that personal or generational responsibilities are recognized; boundaries of relational unit as a whole and subsystems cannot be identified or agreed on; family members are physically endangered or injured or sexually attacked.	1–20: Despair and cynicism are pervasive; there is little attention to the emotional needs of others; there is almost no sense of attachment, commitment, or concern about one another's welfare.

Source: Adapted from Yingling et al. 1998.

and behavior control (Epstein et al. 2003). Table 5.2 gives a fuller description of the dimensions of the MMFF. As there is limited time to meet with the family on the inpatient unit, an abbreviated family assessment with questions derived from the MMFF is helpful. This is illustrated in the following case examples, which use scripted questions from several of the MMFF dimensions.

TABLE 5.2
McMaster Model of Family Functioning

PRESENTING PROBLEM (problems or difficulties identified by the family). "What are you most concerned about? What are the major problems facing your family?" Family discussion of the problems, gathering for each problem, when they first noticed the problem, how have they tried to resolve the problem, and what happened that the problem has not been resolved?

Dimensions

ROLES (recurrent patterns of behavior by which family members fulfill practical and emotional family functioning).

Provision of Resources: How do you divide up the chores? Who does the cooking, grocery shopping, laundry, yard work, care of the car? Are things divided fairly? Does anyone feel overwhelmed? Does anyone feel he or she has too much to do? Do you feel that you get enough help from other members of the family? How are finances organized in your family? Who brings in the money? Are there separate bank accounts? Do the bills get paid? Do you have money troubles? Are you in debt? If so, do you have a plan for paying off your debts? Do you discuss how money is spent? Do the children get an allowance? Do they have to do chores to receive their allowance?

Nurturance and Support: Whom do you go to when you need someone to talk to or when you have a bad day? Is that person helpful? What does the person do that's helpful? What stops you from going to X? When you can't turn to your family, what is it that prevents you?

Sexual Relationship: (Excuse other family members and ask questions of the couple in private.) Are you an affectionate couple? How do the two of you feel about the affectional and sexual aspect of your relationship? Are you having sexual difficulties? When did the difficulties start? Was there a time when your sexual relationship was good? Do you feel satisfied with the affectional and sexual aspect of your relationship? Would you like things to be different; if so, how? Do you both agree or do you see it differently?

Life Skill Development: Who usually oversees the children's education? Who helps the children with school work? Who deals with school issues, attends school meetings? Are the adults able to discuss with each other their careers, changes in jobs?

Maintenance and Management of Family System: Who is involved in major decisions? Who has the final say? Whose opinion is followed if you can't reach an agreement? Where does "the buck stop"?

Role Allocation and Accountability: How do you decide who does each of the jobs in your house? Do you talk about it? Do any of you feel overburdened by your jobs? Are some people doing jobs that they should not be doing? How do you check that jobs get done? Who does that? What do you do if jobs are not getting done?

PROBLEM SOLVING (family's ability to resolve problems to maintain effective family functioning). Includes problems of everyday life (e.g., household repairs, buying an appliance) and emotional problems (e.g., family member angry or sad).

(continued)

TABLE 5.2
McMaster Model of Family Functioning (continued)

Identification: When did you first notice the problem? Who first noticed the problem? Are you the one who notices problems? Who else notices problems?

Communication: When you first notice a problem, what happens? Whom do you tell? Does anyone else notice the problem but not tell anyone?

Development of Alternatives: After you have noticed a problem and communicated about it, do you think about solutions? Who thinks of the plan? Does anyone else have ideas? Do you share them?

Decisions and Actions: How do you decide what to do? Who decides? How do you choose among alternatives?

Monitoring the Action: When you decide on your choice of action, do you follow through? Who does what? Do you usually check to see that things get done after you decide? Who usually checks?

COMMUNICATION (recurrent patterns of how practical and emotional information and messages are exchanged within the family). Three areas of communication are addressed: extent, clarity, and directness.

Extent of Communication: Do people in the family talk much with each other? Who does most of the talking? Can you talk freely to each other, or are you guarded about what you say? What stops you from talking freely to each other?

Clarity of Communication: How did X let you know that? How did you get the message? What is X getting at? What is X telling you? What do you make of what X is saying?

Directness of Communication: Do you feel that others understand you? What happens when they don't? Can you get straight to the point? Do members of the family let you know they have understood what you are trying to say? How do they do that? Do you feel that others understand you? What happens when they don't?

AFFECTIVE RESPONSIVENESS (whether and to what extent family members experience a range of emotions appropriate and in proportion to situations). Do you experience feelings of happiness, joy, sadness, anger, fear? Do you feel that you over-respond with any one emotion? Do you under-respond? Do you think you get angry, depressed, etc., in situations in which others would react differently? Are you concerned about how you respond in some situations?

AFFECTIVE INVOLVEMENT (extent to which family members show a genuine interest in each other). Who cares about what is important to you? What activities and interests are important to you? Is your family supportive of your interests? How do they show their interest? Do they ask you about your activities or hobbies? Do you have a sense that the family cares about what is important to you? How do other family members, including your parents, let you know that they are interested in your activities? Do they show too much interest?

(continued)

TABLE 5.2
McMaster Model of Family Functioning (continued)

Behavior Control (pattern for handling behavior of children and adults in physically dangerous situations). How do you handle discipline in your family? Do you have rules? If so, what are they? Are the rules the same for everyone? Can you give me an example? In which areas are the rules most important in your family? Are the rules clear about how to handle dangerous situations? Can you give me an example of such a situation and the rules you have for it? Is that the same for everyone, or does it vary from person to person? If so, how? Does anyone in the family have a problem with drinking, drugs, violence? Are you concerned about anyone in your family in terms of drinking, drugs, or violence? Are there any particular rules that anyone in the family feels are unfair? Do mother and father agree on the rules? Which rules do you differ on and how? Do you work together as a team in disciplining your children? Tell me how you enforce the rules. Who does the enforcing of the rules? Do children know what to expect if they break a rule? Do parents both enforce the rules? Who is tougher in terms of consequences and punishments? Does that person stick to being tough, or does he or she give in later?

Source: Adapted from Epstein and Bishop 1981, Epstein et al. 2003, and Ryan et al. 2005.

CASE EXAMPLE: AN OVERWHELMED MOTHER AND HER TWO DAUGHTERS

Mary Osbourne, a 45-year-old divorced mother of two teenage daughters, Kisha (17) and Kasandra (13), is admitted with major depression. For the last year, Mary has been the sole caregiver for her 85-year-old mother, who came to live with the family after suffering a hip fracture. Historically, Mary and her mother have had a stormy relationship. Mary's mother was verbally abusive of Mary throughout her childhood and in recent years had rarely seen Mary. Mary's siblings are estranged from their mother because of the mother's verbal abuse of them in childhood. Mary chose to take her mother into her home after the injury, even though Mary had been working two jobs, as a legal secretary during the week and as a restaurant hostess on weekends. Mary's mother died, from complications of hip surgery, two weeks before Mary's admission to the hospital. Mary's current worries include that her younger daughter, Kasandra, is involved with the wrong crowd, defies curfews, skips school, and may be using drugs. Mary is also concerned about her elder daughter, Kisha, who is quiet and withdrawn. Kisha is a devoted daughter and an A student who is planning on becoming a physician. Mary's mother, while living with them, was verbally abusive of both girls. Mary's ex-husband has no contact with the family.

The Resident's Concerns

Dr. Miller, a first-year psychiatric resident, is concerned that Mary, who has been very depressed and preoccupied with feelings of guilt, may become overwhelmed in a family meeting, but Mary wants to confront Kasandra about her disobedient and self-destructive behaviors, and Dr. Miller wants to help Mary resume her role as a strong parent. Dr. Miller knows that she will have just one opportunity to meet with Mary and her daughters together and, in a discussion with her supervisor, questions if a single family meeting will help Mary.

The Supervisor's Response

The supervisor and Dr. Miller establish that the purpose of the family meeting is to assess the family factors that contribute to Mary's depression and to help Mary reestablish herself as an effective parent. Dr. Miller agrees that she must resist being a "cheerleader" for Mary, in case Mary is unable to reach her goal in the family session. The supervisor suggests that Dr. Miller talk with Mary in advance about her expectations for the meeting and antic-ipate how Kasandra will respond to her setting limits. For example, Dr. Miller might ask Mary, "What's the worst that can happen in the meeting? What do you fear? What will it be like for you if Kasandra refuses to obey your rules?" Also Dr. Miller might role play with Mary, acting as Kasandra and becoming belligerent and resisting limits. Dr. Miller expresses doubt that Mary will be able to cope if the daughters show anger at her for not pro-tecting them from their grandmother's verbal abuse. Mary has acknowl-edged not protecting them from their grandmother and wants to apologize to her daughters.

The supervisor comments that the family's coming together to discuss Mary's depression, how the grandmother affected their lives, and the younger daughter's behavior can, in itself, be of great benefit. Focusing on going forward and how things are going to be different will be helpful. The supervisor suggests that Dr. Miller review the MMFF dimension of behavior control for specific questions to ask about behavior problems and difficulties with parenting. Questions from the problem-solving dimension can also help structure the assessment. The supervisor plans to attend the meeting to provide support for Dr. Miller and to intervene if necessary.

The Resident's Intervention

Dr. Miller begins the meeting by orienting the family. She asks each member what she thinks is going to happen in today's meeting. The daughters state that they aren't sure but they want to help their mother. Mary states that she hopes the meeting will help her daughters understand her depression. Dr. Miller explains that she wants to talk about Mary's depression and review other family problems and she lets them know that the meeting will last about one hour.

For each problem the family members identify, Dr. Miller will gather a short history of the problem by asking the following three questions:

1. Have you discussed the problem?
2. How have you tried to resolve the problem?
3. What prevented you from resolving the problem?

These questions gather important information and impose a structure to help move the discussion along in a timely fashion. If the discussion of any detail becomes too lengthy, these questions help the resident stay on track.

Dr. Miller asks Kisha and Kasandra to identify what they are most concerned about.

PROBLEM 1. *The Daughters' Concerns that the Mother Allowed the Grandmother to Be Abusive*

The daughters state that Mary "works herself into a depression" and that they are relieved that it is just the three of them living together again, now that grandmother has passed away. They report that their mother "did everything for her despite how mean and hateful she was." The daughters say that it was upsetting to see how their mother tried to please their grandmother. Kasandra expresses anger toward her mother. "She was such a wimp and took such abuse from her mother!" Kasandra confronts her mother, saying, "Why did you let her be so mean to you? You gave her all your attention and just ignored us!" Mary responds, "It's not an excuse, but I just couldn't stand up to her. I know I should have. I let you both down and I'm so sorry."

Dr. Miller gives the family feedback. "Grandmother was very abusive to all three of you. Mary, you weren't able to intervene on your daughters' behalf, and you feel very sorry that you didn't protect them. Is that right?" The family agrees. Then she asks the three questions.

Have you discussed the problem? The daughters say that they have discussed it between themselves. They report that they repeatedly tried to talk with their mother, but it did no good. Mary tearfully admits again that she just couldn't stand up to her mother, especially since her mother was ill. Dr. Miller asks Kisha for her input. Kisha says, "It was hard to see my mother be beaten down by my grandmother." Kasandra says, "It is frustrating to see my mother, who is usually so strong, not stand up for herself or for us." Mary tearfully apologizes again for allowing her mother to mistreat her daughters. Mary says that the thing she feels most guilty about is not having done more to intervene when her mother was mean to her daughters.

How have you tried to resolve the problem? Kisha and Kasandra report, "We would straighten Grandmother out when she started in on us." Kisha says she would "yell at her to stop picking on our mother. Grandmother was a miserable person." Kasandra says, "I yelled at my mother" for putting up with the grandmother's verbal abuse.

What prevented you from resolving the problem? Both daughters feel angry with their mother for not being able to stop the abuse, but both feel guilty about being angry at her because she is depressed.

Dr. Miller summarizes the presenting problem and gives the family feedback: "All three of you have identified that Mary allowed her mother to verbally abuse all of you. Kasandra and Kisha, you tried to tell your mother how upset you were not only at being verbally abused but also because Mary did nothing to stop the abuse. Mary, you took no action to solve the problem. Also your daughters are both worried about you and feel guilty for being angry with you because they understand that you are depressed. Have I got that right?" Mary and her daughters agree that Dr. Miller understands their problem.

Dr. Miller asks, "How were things among the three of you before Grandmother came to live with you?" All three agree that their family life was good. Mary and her daughters relax as they discuss life before Grandmother came. They recall that the family functioned well and the household ran efficiently. Dr. Miller identified their previous good family functioning as a strength. The family seems pleased to have their pre-Grandmother home life identified as a strength.

Then Dr. Miller asks, "Are there other issues that are problems for your family?"

PROBLEM 2. *The Mother's Concerns regarding Kasandra's Disobedience*

Mary says, "Kasandra has been out of control. She has been breaking curfew and skipping school."

Have you discussed the problem? Mary states that she has talked with Kasandra about her breaking the rules and has tried to reason with her. Dr. Miller asks the following questions from the MMFF dimension of behavior control: "What are the rules in your home? What is the curfew, and what happens if you break the curfew?" Kisha says that they must be home at 9 P.M. on school nights and by 11:30 P.M. on weekends. Kisha relates what happens when Mary punishes Kasandra for coming in late and for skipping school. "Mom grounds her for the weekend, but Kasandra goes out anyway." Dr. Miller asks Mary and Kasandra for their input. Kasandra shrugs her shoulders. Mary says she never had trouble with Kasandra before this school year.

How have you tried to resolve the problem? Mary says, "I've tried to set limits, but it just isn't working. Kasandra basically does what she wants." Mary continues, "I ground Kasandra but I admit I eventually give in to her because she wears me down. I know I should be stronger in disciplining Kasandra but I just haven't been up to the battle." Mary looks at her younger daughter and declares, "But things are going to change. I'm telling you, Kasandra, you will be grounded if you break the curfew or skip school. I mean it." Dr. Miller asks Kasandra for her response. Kasandra says nothing.

Mary then expresses her fear that Kasandra is smoking marijuana. At first Kasandra is defensive and starts raising her voice. Mary counters, "Don't raise your voice to me. I'm your mother and you need to be respectful." Kasandra starts to cry. After a short time, Kasandra apologizes to her mother. Dr. Miller supports Kasandra. "I can see how upset you are and I appreciate that you're on the hot seat. Your mother sounds very worried about you." Kasandra continues crying. Dr. Miller asks Mary to address Kasandra directly. Mary asks Kasandra, "Tell me the truth, have you been smoking marijuana?" Kasandra says that she uses marijuana on weekends. Kisha admits that she knew her sister was smoking marijuana, but didn't want to tell on her and get her in trouble. Mary tells Kasandra that she will not tolerate her using illegal drugs, that Kasandra must come home directly after school, and that she is grounded for the coming weekend. Dr. Miller refocuses the session by asking the third question.

What prevented you from resolving the problem? Mary allows that she just hasn't been able to enforce the rules. "I know I give in, but it's been so hard. I'm really worried about Kasandra." Dr. Miller asks Mary what is going to be different going forward. "What will you do if Kasandra starts pressuring you to let her go out? Are you going to enforce your rules? Do you believe Kasandra when she says she won't smoke marijuana again?" Mary insists that she will enforce the rules. Mary says, "I know my daughters need me to be strong, and before my mother came to live with us, I had no problem in disciplining my girls. Kasandra, I don't know if I believe you when you say you won't smoke marijuana again. You'll have to prove it to me. And you can bet I'll be making sure you abide by rules." Dr. Miller asks the girls if they believe that their mother will follow through on enforcing the rules. Kisha says, "I think my mother is being fair and that it's true that she always made us follow the rules before she got sick." Reluctantly Kasandra agrees, "Mom is being fair and I think she means it."

Dr. Miller gives the family feedback, "As a family, you agree that before Mother became ill, she was a strong mother who would not hesitate to enforce the rules. But over the last months, Mary, since you have been depressed, you've not been able to enforce the rules. Kasandra, you've been skipping school, breaking curfew, and smoking marijuana. Your mother says that you must come directly home after school and you are grounded for the weekend. Kasandra, you have promised your family that you will no longer smoke marijuana and will abide by the rules. Kasandra and Kisha, you both believe that your mother is fair and you will follow her rules. Have I got it right?" The family agrees with Dr. Miller's feedback.

Dr. Miller asks if there are any other problems the family wants to discuss. The family says that they have no other issues. As the meeting comes to a close, Dr. Miller summarizes the meeting, "You are a family with many strengths. You care very much for each other and your family was doing well until your grandmother came to live with you. It was a painful and maddening time for you, daughters, to see your competent mother reduced to tears and intimated by your grandmother. You are angry that your mother couldn't stand up to your grandmother and stop the verbal abuse. Mary, it's been a difficult time for you as you have suffered with depression, and it's good that you are feeling stronger. I know you have many feelings of sadness and anger about your relationship with your mother, but I hope you can find peace knowing you did all you could for her in her last months. You've been able to set limits with Kasandra in this meeting and will enforce her punishment of coming home after school and not going out this weekend. It's important to remember how strong your family is and how much you care for one another." The family agrees with Dr. Miller's summary and says the family meeting has been helpful. They discuss coming back for a full family assessment, but the family declines. Finally, Dr. Miller tells them that they are a very nice family and wishes them luck. Kasandra stands up and hugs her mother. Kisha joins in the hug and all three are smiling as the meeting ends.

GARF Assessment

Using the GARF scale Dr. Miller calculates an overall family relational functioning rating of 49:

1. Interactional problem solving = 40. Family life was totally disrupted when Mary's mother came to live with them. The family was unsuccessful in solving the problem of Mary's mother's verbal abuse of the family members. There is also painful conflict around Kasandra's curfew violations and smoking marijuana. Kasandra breaks the rules and defies her mother's attempts to set firm limits.

2. Organization = 42. Mary's mother usurped Mary's power as an effective head of the household. Mary placated and tried to please her mother, and so was unable to stop her mother's verbal attacks on herself and her daughters.

3. Emotional climate = 65. Mary and her daughters have remained warm and caring of each other. Despite Mary's mother's tirades,

which disrupted the emotional climate of their family, Mary and her daughters continue to express their concern for each other.

Lessons Learned

The goals of this abbreviated family assessment have been met. The structured family meeting allowed a history of the presenting problem to be reviewed. The family and Dr. Miller established the impact of the grandmother on Mary and the impact of Mary's depression on Kasandra, a three-generational pattern of family factors influencing Mary's presentation of depression. Understanding these impacts was crucial in helping Dr. Miller and the family work collaboratively. Dr. Miller used questions from the MMFF behavior control dimension to gain an understanding of Kasandra's behavior problems. She used the GARF to describe the family's overall level of functioning. The assessment is a success, as the family is able to discuss and reach some resolution of their major problems. The case example of Mary Osbourne and her daughters illustrates how a single session with a family can be beneficial.

CASE EXAMPLE: MR. AND MS. GREEN
(FROM CHAPTER 2) DON'T GET DIVORCED

Ms. Green was admitted to the hospital with major depression, recurrent. Dr. Stevens, who had initially met with the couple (see Chapter 2) meets with them again on the inpatient unit. Ms. Green has had difficulty talking with her husband about her depression and has habitually turned to her mother for support. She continues to be fearful that her husband wants a divorce.

The Resident's Concerns

Dr. Stevens is anxious about how to proceed. How will she help Mr. and Ms. Green with their communication about her depression and suicidal thinking? Dr. Stevens is surprised at the persistence of Ms. Green's belief that Mr. Green wants a divorce. Dr. Stevens thought that Mr. Green's reassurance in their previous couples' session would have allayed Ms. Green's fears. Dr. Stevens is also concerned about budgeting her time so that she is able to adequately address the family problems as well as medication management and posthospital planning.

The Supervisor's Response

The supervisor points out that the purpose of the meeting is to more fully assess and possibly improve the communication between Mr. and Ms. Green. Specifically, the goal of the meeting is to help the couple understand their lack of communication about Ms. Green's depression and chronic suicidal thoughts, understand why Ms. Green turns to her mother for nurturance and support rather than to her husband, and to identify Mr. Green's commitment to the marriage. The supervisor advises Dr. Stevens to pay particular attention to the orientation, the development of the list of problems, and giving feedback to the couple. The supervisor reminds Dr. Stevens that she doesn't have to help the couple solve major issues in the assessment, that offering encouragement and support to the couple for discussing painful subjects will in itself be helpful. Dr. Stevens can say to the couple, "I know it is very difficult and frightening to talk about suicidal thoughts."

The Resident's Intervention

Dr. Stevens begins the family session with an orientation to identify what Mr. and Ms. Green think will be addressed and accomplished in the meeting. "It's nice to see you both again. I'd like to start by asking each of you what you expect we will do in the meeting today."

Dr. Stevens gives a clear synopsis of what is said as well as outlining her expectations of the meeting: "Mr. Green, you thought we were going to discuss your wife's depression, and Ms. Green, you weren't sure what we were going to do today. OK, let me tell you what I think we can do in this meeting. We'll meet for an hour and I want to make certain that we discuss each of your concerns. I want to gain a greater understanding of how you function as a couple. We know that how a couple functions affects each of you individually, and what is going on with each of you individually affects the other person. I'll be asking a variety of questions and I'll let you know what I'm thinking, so please correct me if you think I'm getting the wrong impression. I also want to make sure we discuss Ms. Green's progress in the hospital and answer any questions about the hospitalization or posthospital plans. I want to make sure that at the end of our time together today, we have a better understanding of the issues facing your family. Does this plan for today's meeting sound reasonable?" Dr. Stevens obtains an agreement from the couple before proceeding.

Dr. Stevens asks Mr. and Ms. Green to identify their concerns. Usually, but not always, the family will identify the patient's illness and current hospitalization as their most pressing concern. In this case, Ms. Green's depression and suicidal ideation are the presenting problem. Dr. Stevens ensures that both Mr. and Ms. Green give their perspectives on this issue and agree to her assessment of the problem.

The next task is to develop the list of problems. Dr. Stevens develops the list by asking the couple, "Are there other issues that are problems for your family?" For each problem identified, Dr. Stevens gathers a short history by asking the three questions

1. Have you discussed the problem?
2. How have you tried to resolve the problem?
3. What prevented you from resolving the problem?

PROBLEM 1. *Fear of Divorce*

Ms. Green speaks first. Despite Mr. Green's assurance in their initial session that he wants to remain in the marriage, her biggest concern is that her husband truly wants a divorce. Ms. Green acknowledges that he says he doesn't want a divorce, but she states that their marriage is in trouble.

Since our last session, have you discussed the problem? No. Dr. Stevens asks Ms. Green why she hasn't discussed her concerns with her husband. Ms. Green answers that she is fearful of what he will say.

How have you tried to resolve the problem? Rather than talk with Mr. Green about her fear of his leaving her, Ms. Green tries to please Mr. Green and appear happy. Dr. Stevens asks Mr. Green if he was aware that his wife continued to fear that they will divorce. Mr. Green repeats that he had had no idea and that he wants the marriage to work. He is surprised that his wife pretends to be happy in order to please him.

What prevented you from resolving the problem? Ms. Green replies that her husband becomes upset and withdraws when she tries to talk with him about anything unpleasant. Mr. Green responds that it is hard for him to talk about feelings and that he is aware that they don't communicate about problems.

PROBLEM 2. *Communication*

They agree that they have a problem with communication and cannot discuss important issues. *Have you discussed the problem?* No. They agree that they are unable to discuss Ms. Green's illness, especially her suicidal thoughts, or any other problems. *How have you tried to resolve the issue?* Ms. Green says that when she tries to talk with her husband about her depression, he becomes nervous and tells her not to worry. *What prevented you from resolving the problem?* Ms. Green says because her husband won't talk about anything unpleasant, she turns to her mother. Mr. Green admits that, because it is hard for him to talk about unpleasant thoughts and feelings, he tends to back away from discussion about his wife's depression. He adds that he tries to cheer her up by telling her not to worry and that he doesn't know what else to say. Dr. Stevens asks the couple to discuss the issue further. Mr. Green asks his wife why she turns to her mother. Ms. Green replies that she can openly discuss her depression with her mother. Dr. Stevens asks Ms. Green how her mother is of help. Ms. Green describes her mother as calm and says she helps her to cope by distracting her. Ms. Green wishes her husband could be there for her, like her mother. Mr. Green agrees that his wife needs to talk about her depression and that he needs to learn to discuss it with her.

Dr. Stevens asks Mr. Green what it's like for him to know that his wife has suicidal thoughts. He replies that it is frightening. Dr. Stevens asks if he thinks his wife understands how he feels, how very difficult it is for him to know that she has thoughts of wanting to die and yet he doesn't know how to help her? He responds, "Not really." He adds that he doesn't know how to reassure his wife and is afraid that if he doesn't say the right thing it will make her worse. Dr. Stevens asks Ms. Green to respond. Ms. Green says that she has never thought about how upsetting it is for her husband. In discussing their unsuccessful efforts to communicate, the couple begins to understand how and where their communication breaks down. Dr. Stevens summarizes and gives them feedback on their problem with communication.

"Ms. Green, when your attempts to gain reassurance from your husband fail, you turn to your mother. Mr. Green, you want to be helpful, but because you cannot tolerate discussing unpleasant issues, you withdraw and you both are unable to communicate and resolve this problem."

PROBLEM 3. Mr. Green's Lack of Understanding of His Wife's Illness

Have you discussed the problem? Ms. Green says that she has tried to discuss her condition with her husband; she thinks he doesn't understand her depression. Mr. Green agrees that he does need to learn more and admits, "I guess I don't want to believe it."

How have you tried to resolve the problem? Ms. Green has given her husband written material on depression and has asked him to accompany her to her outpatient appointments.

What prevented you from resolving the problem? Ms. Green replies that her husband is always "too busy." Ms. Green asks Dr. Stevens to tell her husband about depression. Dr. Stevens provides psychoeducation. Ms. Green asks her husband if he will accompany her to her next appointment. He agrees to and repeats that he wants to be supportive. At this point the resident asks if there are other problems facing the couple.

PROBLEM 4. Mr. Green's Belief That His Wife's Mother Is Too Involved in Their Marriage

Have you discussed the problem? The couple reply that they have.

How have you tried to resolve the problem? Ms. Green says she has repeatedly explained to her husband that her mother is a major source of support that she needs. She wishes her husband were more understanding of her need to have a close relationship with her mother. She does not think her mother interferes in their marriage. Mr. Green sees things very differently. He insists that he understands and supports his wife's having a close relationship with her mother, but he does not like the fact that she is closer to her mother than she is to him. He also states that her mother has too much to say about their marriage. (Dr. Stevens chooses to ignore this comment, keeping to the problem-solving focus of the interview.)

What prevented you from resolving the problem? The couple's previous attempts to solve the problem resulted in circular arguments in which they would repeatedly restate their own positions. They stick steadfastly to their individual positions, unable to acknowledge any valid aspects of the other person's perspective on the problem. Dr. Stevens says, "I understand that you have very different positions on this issue and aren't able at this point to compromise, so for now you'll have to agree to disagree on this issue." The resident then adds the problem and the couple's different perspectives to the list of problems. If the couple enters into treatment, these problems will be addressed in greater depth.

As the meeting comes to an end, Dr. Stevens reviews Ms. Green's progress in the hospital and addresses questions about her medications. It has been decided that she will stay in the hospital two more days. Dr. Stevens reviews a summary of the presenting problem and the additional items on their list of problems. They agree to another meeting before Ms. Green's discharge to continue the assessment.

Dr. Stevens gives the Greens an overall GARF rating of 41.

1. Interactional problem solving = 30. The couple presents initially with major problems in communication and as a result cannot resolve Ms. Green's fear that her husband wants a divorce. Similarly, the couple have been unable to discuss Ms. Green's illness and the issue of Ms. Green's mother's status as sole confidante of Ms. Green.

2. Organization = 35. Ms. Green turns to her mother instead of her husband to help her cope and manage her illness. Mr. Green considers his wife's mother to be overly involved in their marriage.

3. Emotional climate = 58. While the couple has problems, they care deeply for each other. They have however, stopped spending time together and no longer share common leisure activities. Mr. Green is withdrawn emotionally from his wife because she has turned to her mother for support that he does not know how to provide. The couple's intimacy and sexual relationship have deteriorated.

Assessment of the Greens' Family Functioning

During the third and final meeting with the Greens in the hospital, Dr. Stevens completes a full family assessment using the MMFF. She then reviews the list of problems with Mr. and Ms. Green. They all agree on the following problems:

1. Fear of divorce: The couple has not been sexually intimate in several months; Ms. Green cites this fact and her husband's apparent indifference to her turning to her mother as proof that he wants a divorce.
2. Communication: Ms. Green is unclear and indirect in her communication style. This means that Mr. Green does not understand her intent and ignores her. Ms. Green interprets this behavior as a lack of caring, which again reinforces her turning to her mother for support. Their communication style impedes the resolution of their emotional problems.
3. In the dimension of affective involvement, they have identified that they do not spend as much time together as they would like.
4. Mr. Green's lack of understanding of his wife's illness.

Dr. Stevens asks the couple if they want to enter treatment. She explains that family treatment is the action part of family work and will focus on negotiating, working on problems, and making changes.

Family Treatment

After Ms. Green's discharge from the hospital, Dr. Stevens has two treatment sessions with the couple. She asks them which issue they want to address first. They identify that they do not spend quality time together. They agree that they have enjoyed reestablishing their practice of playing board games after dinner, as agreed upon in their initial meeting with Dr. Stevens. They then agree exactly how this will happen each evening: while Mr. Green clears the table and washes up after the evening meal, Ms. Green will set up the Scrabble board in the living room. They agree to alternate weeks for clearing up after dinner and choosing which game they will play. Dr. Stevens adds that this is a good time to connect with each other but not a time to discuss problems.

For the second half of this session, Dr. Stevens wants to help the couple improve their communication. She chooses to do this by asking the couple to negotiate changes in the following way. She asks Mr. and Ms. Green to turn their chairs to face each other and then asks Ms. Green to tell her husband what she needs from him. "I need you to listen to me when I'm upset and frightened by my thoughts." At Dr. Stevens's prompting, Ms. Green continues, "I want you to acknowledge what I'm saying to you and not prematurely reassure me that everything is O.K. and not to worry." Mr. Green agrees that he will do this. Dr. Stevens asks Mr. Green to tell his wife any concerns or fears he has about having her talk openly with him about her illness. Mr. Green says, "I need you to tell me when you start having suicidal thoughts and not go to your mother." Dr. Stevens intervenes, suggesting that Mr. Green check in with Ms. Green on a regular basis about how she is feeling rather than waiting until things deteriorate to the point where she is feeling suicidal. The couple acknowledge that this makes sense. They decide that when they are spending time before dinner sharing how their day has been, Mr. Green will ask Ms. Green how she is feeling. Ms. Green will tell Mr. Green if she needs to talk with him. Dr. Stevens suggests that, when they are discussing Ms. Green's feelings, Mr. Green let his wife know if he starts feeling overwhelmed. The couple agree to keep their conversations about her depression to 15 minutes. Also, if Ms. Green is feeling suicidal and needs to talk beyond 15 minutes, she will contact her therapist or psychiatrist, not her mother.

In the final session of family treatment, the couple report that they have been talking and checking in with each other. Ms. Green has been able to tell her husband when she has had some fleeting suicidal thoughts. Mr. Green was able to listen to her and avoid prematurely reassuring her. Dr. Stevens congratulates them on this important progress. She then reviews the list of problems one by one, and the couple report that they feel that things are much improved and that they are satisfied with their progress in treatment. When Dr. Stevens asks them about Ms. Green's mother's involvement, they insist that since Ms. Green has been able to talk to him, Mr. Green no longer feels threatened by her relationship with her mother. The couple is more tentative when discussing their difficulties with sexual intimacy. They both say that overall things are better and that they believe their sexual intimacy will improve over time. Dr. Stevens observes that the couple is hesitant in discussing the sexual aspect of their relationship. They give vague answers but insist that they are pleased with the intimate aspect of their relationship. They both think that because things are better, they don't need to continue in family treatment.

Dr. Stevens reviews their treatment successes: improvements in communication, understanding of illness, spending more quality time together, Mr. Green's ability to support his wife when she needs to talk, improved sexual intimacy, and agreement that Ms. Green's mother's is not too involved. Importantly, Dr. Stevens reminds the couple that while all families have problems that arise from time to time, they have learned how to better resolve problems on their own. The couple agree that they have a better understanding of how to negotiate and resolve issues. Dr. Stevens supports their positive attitude and tells them it has been a pleasure to work with them.

Lessons Learned

The goals of the family assessment and family treatment have been met: Dr. Stevens used the MMFF dimensions of roles and communication to guide her exploration of the couple's problems. The first two meetings consisted of an abbreviated assessment in which only the highlights were addressed. This was successful, and the family asked for a full assessment, then family treatment. Before beginning the treatment phase, Dr. Stevens explained and secured an agreement from the couple that they indeed wanted to enter family treatment. She then helped the couple negotiate and resolve their major problems. Dr. Stevens listened to the couple when they indicated that their sexual intimacy was improved; she did not press the couple to continue treatment, even though she suspected that it would yield further improvement.

SUMMARY

A full family assessment is, of course, superior to an abbreviated family assessment. However, time constraints on a busy inpatient service necessitate the development of an abbreviated assessment model. In an abbreviated assessment, the resident can establish an alliance with the family and obtain a short history of each of the family problems. In a full assessment, a detailed history of family functioning can be obtained and a comprehensive problem list established. A full assessment can be followed by formal treatment, with the family's agreement.

In the case example of Mary Osbourne and her daughters, the abbreviated assessment on the inpatient unit was sufficient to reestablish the family's prior functioning. The Osbourne family was confident that a full assessment was not necessary. In the case of the Greens, an abbreviated assessment was followed by a full family assessment and treatment.

A family assessment, full or abbreviated, provides the resident with an understanding of how family factors may contribute to the patient's illness and/or hospitalization. The abbreviated assessment illustrated in this chapter is based on the McMaster model of family assessment. The GARF, another assessment tool, described in the DSM IV-TR, also provides the busy resident with a way to assess the families of their patients.

CHAPTER SIX

Managing a Family Meeting

Successful management of a family meeting requires specific strategies for intervening with "challenging" families. Five common mistakes that residents make in managing family meetings are discussed. These mistakes are: (1) not recognizing the family's strengths, (2) avoiding the hostile family, (3) just winging it, (4) poor time management, and (5) believing the physician can solve the family's problems. Strategies to manage challenging family members are presented. These strategies are: setting limits with the dominant powerbroker, the monopolizer, the angry family member, and the chaotic family, and engaging the silent member. The use of role-playing as a teaching tool is suggested. A case example illustrates how to manage a volatile family meeting and set limits with the monopolizer and the angry, out-of-control member.

One of the first tasks when meeting with a family is to understand the "culture" of the family. Every family has its own set of rules and beliefs, which may not be obvious but may greatly influence the family's willingness to work with the treatment team. These beliefs can include a distrust of medications, belief that prayer heals, or the invocation of spirits and communication with ancestors. Beliefs and ways of interacting and expressing conflict can also vary widely by sociocultural group. How emotion is expressed, for example, can influence a family's discussion of conflictual issues. A display of great emotion may be needed in some families to illustrate the seriousness of a situation. Deference to older family members in Asian cultures and emotional constriction in some northern European cultures can interfere with open acknowledgment and discussion of conflicts. When leading a family meeting, the resident may ask the family to educate him or her about the family's ways of handling problems, expressing feelings, and so forth (Dyche and Zayas 1995). More obvious differences occur across sociocultural groups, and an open acknowledgment of these differences between the treating physician and the family can clarify areas of disagreement and help promote a working alliance with the physician. There are many varieties of family beliefs, and it is important that these beliefs and cultural norms not be mislabeled as pathological.

Some families are referred to as "difficult" by members of a treatment team. A "difficult" family is defined as one that presents a particular challenge to these team members. Such families typically include one or more "difficult" family members, who may (1) dominate the session, (2) talk over and answer for other members, (3) be angry or challenging, (4) be out of control, or (5) be silent and nonparticipatory. Supervisors should not underestimate the level of anxiety and distress that residents can experience when dealing with an affectively charged family. It is worthwhile for the supervisor to meet with the resident before each meeting and carefully review these concerns.

"Difficult" or even hostile behavior does not necessarily indicate that the family is dysfunctional. The vast majority of families are not dysfunctional or pathological; most are "basically and potentially competent" (Mohr, Lafuz, and Mohr 2000). An understanding of the "culture" of the family and the family's point of view are the first requisites to successfully working with families. The most common mistake physicians make in working with patient's families is to avoid families that are displaying hostile behavior. Four other common mistakes that physicians make are not recognizing the family's strengths, "just winging it" instead of properly preparing for a meeting, poor management of time during the meeting, and the belief that the physician can solve the family's problems. In this chapter, several scenarios will be described that use scripted strategies for intervening with "difficult" families. Supervisor-led role-playing with residents is an excellent method for learning how to implement these strategies. This chapter's case example illustrates how to manage a meeting with a monopolizer, an out-of-control adolescent, and a silent member.

COMMON MISTAKES
Not Recognizing the Family's Strengths

Physicians are trained to identify pathology, so they often focus exclusively on a family's problems. While families have weaknesses, they also have strengths. Acknowledging family strengths contributes to improved patient outcome in several ways. First, it helps to establish an alliance between the physician and the family. The physician can begin the meeting by simply thanking the family for coming and acknowledging any distance or other obstacles they might have traversed to attend the meeting. When the physician expresses this sentiment directly to the family, family members tend to relax and become more open and honest. This greater comfort with the doctor makes it easier for them to become actively involved in the patient's treatment and for the physician to work with them in this endeavor.

Second, supporting the family's efforts to be positive and to focus on problem solving enhances the family's strengths and sets the tone for future healthy interactions rather than assigning blame, being critical, or focusing on pathology. Recognizing the family's capabilities also fosters the attitude that treatment will be a collaboration among the patient, the physician, and the family. The physician should acknowledge and support any effort that a family member makes to gather information pertinent to their loved one's illness and treatment. For example, in a family session, the mother of an adolescent patient shares detailed information she has obtained from the Internet which she believes proves that her daughter has bipolar disorder. The physician gives positive recognition of the mother's efforts and obvious caring about her daughter and inquires, "Can you explain why you think your daughter has bipolar disorder?" The mother rejoins, "Well, this article describes my daughter exactly! I was also speaking with a friend whose daughter has bipolar disorder, and she agrees with me." The physician might respond, "That's really great that you have been actively researching information. Can you tell me more about your observations of your daughter's behaviors which leads you to believe that she has bipolar disorder?" After listening to the mother for several minutes, the physician summarizes, "I agree that the behaviors you've described sound very similar to those of someone with bipolar disorder. Before making any diagnosis, however, we will gather some other important information, such as prior medical records, results of lab tests, and information from school. We want to be very thorough." The physician has praised the mother's efforts, taken her observations seriously, and incorporated this information into the diagnostic process. This has encouraged the family to be active, future oriented, and solution focused. Such an attitude on the part of the family will be helpful to the patient on discharge.

Third, acknowledging strengths is helpful because it can reframe for the physician family behaviors and attitudes that physicians are taught to see as psychopathology. The classic example is the "overbearing, overinvolved" mother. Another way of thinking about the mother's behavior is to understand that her behavior also reflects a deep commitment and concern for her child. The physician can point out both the strength and the weakness of the mother's position. For example, "Ms. Delmonico, I recognize your strong commitment and advocacy for your son. However, your intention to be helpful is getting lost in the emotional intensity of the message." Acknowledging the mother's strength allows the physician to ally with the mother while helping her reduce her high level of emotional intensity.

Finally, the physician must remember that the stress of hospitalization of a family member often shows families at their worst. At times of stress, some families become resilient and cope well and others come apart at their weak points. The knowledgeable physician can help families develop resilience by fostering their coping skills. Family resilience is enhanced by helping the family remain cohesive and supportive of each other and supporting clear and direct communication, which in turn facilitates good problem solving. These coping skills are useful all the time but are essential in times of adversity.

Avoiding the Hostile Family

Most families of psychiatric inpatients have been on the frontlines providing care, support, and advocacy for their mentally ill family member. They typically spend hours with the patient in emergency rooms and in hospital admissions offices, trying to secure treatment for their loved one. These families are with the ill family member before admission and at discharge, yet often they do not have adequate access to the treatment team, especially the physician. An angry or distraught family may, unfortunately, have been ignored or mistreated by the mental health system in the past. These families can also have many strengths, which unfortunately can be overlooked in the crisis of the admission and the hospitalization. As discussed above, being mindful of and looking for strengths can be very helpful to the family, the patient, and the treatment team and creates the foundation of a good working alliance.

Family members often are angry and upset because of feelings of helplessness and are on edge and not at their best when interacting with members of the treatment team. The distraught family member usually calms down when the physician takes the time to gently remind the family that he or she is trying to be of help and to understand their concerns. Not taking the time to speak with a hostile family member can exacerbate the family's anger generally. The hostile family member is not likely to go away. Most important, ignoring the family is not beneficial for the patient.

Efforts to protect patient confidentiality can create problems for families and the treatment team. While patient confidentiality law ensures protection of the patient's privacy, it has had the unintended result of erecting barriers between concerned family members and the patient's treatment team. Family members who telephone the hospital may hear the following, "Because of patient confidentiality, I can't confirm that Mr. Jones is a patient in this hospital." A family member, who has finally gotten the patient admitted to the hospital, having spent hours waiting with the patient in the hospital emergency room, may feel outraged to encounter this kind of response from the hospital staff. Members of the treatment team need to recognize how stressful this kind of experience is for families and to be compassionate, even toward the "difficult family member." Hospital staff are in a particularly awkward situation if the patient has not yet signed a release of information form or has refused to sign one. A physician may be on the phone or in the presence of a family member but legally prevented from discussing the patient. However, it is unwise to ignore or rebuff a hostile family even if the patient has not authorized release of information. Doing so can result in complaints and even litigation. It helps to explain to the family member, "I understand how very frustrating and upsetting it must be not to be able to get information about Mr. Jones, but because of the law of patient confidentiality, I, unfortunately, can't give you any information or even acknowledge that Mr. Jones is a patient. However, I can listen to your concerns and you can give me any information that you would like me to have." Generally speaking, patients should be encouraged to sign a release of information, so that their family can be involved. If the patient is reluctant to have the family involved, discussing the patient's concerns and the physician's expectations of family involvement can be reassuring and facilitate the signing of the release form.

"Just Winging It"

The physician who plunges ahead with a family meeting, trusting and hoping that what needs to be discussed will materialize, usually finds that the meeting fails to address some important issues. The result of giving little thought or preparation to a family meeting is usually that the majority of the time is spent exploring the first issues identified by the family and others are never raised. The resident should identify important issues before the session and should bring them up if they do not surface otherwise during the meeting. Although a thorough discussion of one or two problems can be helpful to the family, much of what needs to be discussed can be missed and the resident will thus have no overall understanding of the family. The management of the family meeting is critical, because with inpatients, there may be only one meeting with the family in which to discuss the history of the presenting illness, important family issues, the course of hospitalization, and posthospital planning.

Poor Management of Time

Without a structure to the family meeting, there may be difficulty managing time. At the beginning of the family session, it is often helpful for the physician to explain, "We'll be meeting for approximately one hour. I'll keep an eye on the time, so that everyone has an opportunity to discuss their concerns." If the physician fails to manage the time, the meeting may run overtime in the attempt to cover the major issues or it may end before important problems have been discussed. In these days of managed care and shortened hospital stays, learning good management of time is essential. In addition to assuring that the anticipated important problems are addressed, time also needs to be allocated to explore sensitive issues that may come up unexpectedly. When the family is asked about painful subjects that they have previously treated as "taboo" and not open for discussion, modeling open and honest discussion of these issues is helpful. The physician may even point this out with a statement like, "I know it's very difficult to discuss this issue, but this may be just the time, while John is in the hospital and your family and John have our support."

The Physician's Belief that He or She Can Solve the Family's Problems

It is important to be positive and hopeful for the family's success in resolving their problems but also to be realistic and understand that change is difficult. From the family's perspective, they may already be "doing the best that they can," and although families want relief from their suffering and resolution of their problems, making long-term behavioral change can be difficult, as families resist changes in their homeostatic patterns of living and interacting.

The resident can facilitate a meeting with the patient and family in order to identify family problems. However, the resident needs to be mindful that even when he or she provides the family with a neutral and supportive environment and works with them to identify problems, ultimately it is the family who is responsible for making a commitment to treatment and putting forth their best efforts to solve their problems. In a common scenario, one family member is not ready to change and the others want to change. Such a family system can be understood as resisting change, and whatever efforts the resident makes will most likely be unsuccessful. A resident will often mistakenly persevere in trying to make the family understand why changes should occur. A more therapeutic position is for the resident to state to the family: "Change is hard and requires a commitment from all of you. It seems that at this time not all of you are ready to make changes. If in the future you want to work on these issues, please call me and set up an appointment. Good luck to all of you."

SETTING LIMITS

A family meeting provides a safe, neutral environment in which a family can discuss its concerns. The psychiatrist provides this opportunity for families by managing the family meeting and setting limits if family members become too heated. A successful meeting may depend on the psychiatrist's ability to control the dialogue, set limits, and direct the meeting toward realistic goals. Yalom, a teacher of group therapy, provides invaluable step-by-step interventions that script how to give constructive feedback and set appropriate limits with group members who are engaging in problematic behaviors (1993). His interventions can be adapted for use with families. We describe a two-pronged approach in which the psychiatrist acknowledges positive contributions the family member has made to the session, focusing on the family member's "intention" to be helpful, then explains the effect of the family member's negative behavior. It is important to make the distinction between the person's intention and the unhelpful behavior. "Stroke, stroke, push" is a useful phrase with which to conceptualize this process. First, the therapist "strokes" the family member by giving credit for the efforts and identifying the intention as helpful then "pushes" the family member, setting a limit and giving feedback about the problematic behavior or attitude. Residents may ask, "What do I do if I think the family member is intentionally trying to be hurtful with negative behavior or statements?" It is wise to give the family member the benefit of the doubt and assume that he or she is trying to be helpful. At the very least, this will allow the family member to be engaged more easily and feel heard and thus be more prepared to accept feedback. Furthermore, a family member who feels shamed and humiliated will be unlikely to accept negative feedback. No matter how skillful the intervention, negative feedback always hurts. The two-pronged approach helps the family member be less defensive, enhances his or her ability to hear the feedback, and ultimately sets the stage for change.

Setting limits is necessary with the dominant powerbroker, the monopolizer, the angry and out-of-control family member, and the chaotic family. The dominant powerbroker seeks to neutralize the influence of the therapist and tries to control the session. The monopolizer talks incessantly, interrupts others, and is usually driven by anxiety. The dominant powerbroker and the monopolizer can be, but aren't necessarily, one and the same. Regardless, they must not be allowed to take over the meeting. If a resident fails to neutralize the powerbroker or the monopolizing family member's challenging and disruptive behaviors, the family will accurately conclude that the resident is intimidated and will perceive the resident as ineffective. It can be especially difficult for the young, inexperienced resident to successfully set limits with an older family member, as the resident's age, personal maturity, and life experience can influence credibility (Simon 1989). Early on and throughout the session when necessary, the resident must intervene respectfully but firmly.

Another difficult family member is the silent, nonparticipatory member. The resident should encourage the quiet family member to speak but not get into a struggle, trying too hard to get him or her to participate. Check in with the quiet member throughout the meeting and continue to invite him or her to participate.

The following scripted responses illustrate how best to manage these various types of family members.

The Dominant Powerbroker

Positive statement of intention: "Mr. Stevenson, you have shared many of your concerns and have worked hard in this meeting."

Setting the limit: "Why don't we let other people carry the ball for a while? We should hear from others at this point." If the dominant behavior continues despite the intervention, the resident makes a stronger intervention.

Positive statement of intention: "Mr. Stevenson, I know you're trying to help."

Setting the stronger limit: "But you must stop and let others contribute to the meeting. I think that sometimes, because you have strong opinions and have a lot to say, others are reluctant to share what they are feeling or thinking." Throughout the meeting, the resident should ask Mr. Stevenson to stop if he continues to interrupt the meeting.

The Monopolizer

Positive statement of intention: "Mrs. Matthews, you've tried to help others address some very important concerns and you've been reaching out to everyone."

Setting the limit: "But I think other members need to step up to the plate now and answer for themselves." If Mrs. Matthews continues to talk over others, answering for them, and ignores the intervention, the resident makes a stronger intervention.

Positive statement of intention: "Mrs. Matthews, you've worked hard in this meeting. I know you are trying to help."

Setting stronger limit: "But you need to allow others to share their concerns." The resident then addresses the family, "Does this happen at home? Does Mom answer for everyone?" The family will probably say yes. If so, the resident asks, "Mrs. Matthews, are you aware that you answer for everyone?" The resident can ask the family, "Have you talked about Mom's answering for everyone?" Again, the resident is careful not to shame the mother, saying, "You mean to be helpful, but it's more helpful when everyone takes responsibility and speaks for himself or herself."

The Angry or Challenging Member

Positive statement of intention: "I can see that you're angry and upset and this meeting has been very difficult."

Setting the limit: "But it's hard for me to think about the good points that you are making when you constantly challenge and interrupt me. It's hard to get past your hostile statements." If the family member continues to be angry and challenging despite the intervention, the resident makes a stronger intervention.

Positive statement of intention: "I'm trying to understand your position."

Setting the limit: "But your yelling at me makes it difficult for me to understand where you're coming from."

Stronger limit setting: "If you can't stop yelling, I'll have to end the meeting."

The Silent or Nonparticipating Member

Positive statement of intention: "I don't want to put you on the spot, but I did want to check in with you. I notice you've been listening to everyone today. People who are quiet and are good listeners can usually offer a valuable perspective on what's happening around them."

Setting the limit: "I'm wondering if you could share some of your observations in today's family meeting."

The Chaotic and Out-of-Control Family

Positive statement of intention: "I know this meeting is very upsetting to you all."

Setting the limit: "But everyone must settle down and stop yelling and cursing because we aren't getting anywhere."

Stronger limit setting: "If you can't stop fighting, I'll have to stop the meeting." If the family continues to be out of control, the resident should not hesitate to stop the meeting. If necessary, the resident should stand up and state that the meeting is over. Where appropriate, the resident can offer, "When you are able to participate in a meeting, please call me, but for today, the meeting is over." The resident should escort the family out of the room. If they won't leave, the resident should exit the room. Holding the meeting in a private room on the inpatient unit allows the resident to leave more easily.

ROLE-PLAYING

For residents meeting as a group for supervision, participation in role-plays can provide opportunities to try out different interventions. Supervisor-led role-plays proceed as follows: Each resident takes a turn at being the therapist of a simulated family, composed of other residents. The therapist resident begins to work with the simulated family as they portray a challenging family scenario. When the therapist resident is stumped, the residents who are observing are asked to make suggestions as to what intervention should occur. The resident who makes a suggestion then assumes the role of therapist. Similarly, when the supervisor makes a suggestion, the supervisor takes on the role. Within a single simulated family session, the therapist can change several times as the residents make suggestions and become the therapist. This exercise leads to lively exchanges and provides residents with practical experience. Residents enjoy role-plays and learn from observing their supervisor as the therapist in these simulations.

CASE EXAMPLE: THE EXPLOSIVE FAMILY

Donald Rizzo, a 16-year-old male, is admitted to the hospital's adolescent unit with depressive symptoms, passive suicidal ideation, alcohol abuse, and use of marijuana. Donald has appeared before Family Court charged with possession of marijuana and alcohol, and the judge has ordered him to have a psychiatric evaluation. Donald is suspended from high school. When his parents attempt to set limits for him, he threatens to run away from home. His 9-year-old sister, Lily, is doing well both in school and at home. Notably, Donald's father has a history of substance abuse. Dr. Chou, a second-year psychiatric resident, is meeting with Donald, who tells her that his father is a hypocrite because his father "says he's in recovery but continues to drink and then punishes me for drinking." The next day, Mr. Rizzo calls and insists that Dr. Chou meet with the family right away. Dr. Chou arranges a meeting for the following morning.

The Resident's Concerns

Dr. Chou is very concerned about the potential for Donald and his father to get into a heated argument and is anxious about intervening if the family meeting gets out of control. What if Donald loses control, threatens his father, or storms out of the meeting? Dr. Chou anticipates Mr. Rizzo's raising his voice and lecturing Donald. Dr. Chou is concerned that Donald will confront his father about his drinking; if he does, is it appropriate to question Mr. Rizzo about his drinking, especially because Mr. Rizzo is not her patient and has told the treatment team that he is in recovery? Dr. Chou dreads the family meeting.

The Supervisor's Response

The supervisor and Dr. Chou discuss the goals of the meeting. The parents want Donald to obey their rules, stop drinking, stop smoking marijuana, and attend school. Dr. Chou and the supervisor agree with the parents' goals, but also want to support Donald in respectfully confronting his father on his drinking. They also want to help the family have a successful discussion and begin work on resolving problems.

The supervisor asks Dr. Chou directly, "What are your fears about meeting with this family?" Dr. Chou says that the most difficult aspect of the meeting for her will be the probability of having to confront and set limits with Donald's father. She states that in her Asian culture it is highly irregular for a woman to confront the male head of household and, while she believes she can intervene appropriately with Mr. Rizzo, it will make her very anxious. Dr. Chou also openly acknowledges her fear that the family session will get out of control, especially if Donald confronts his father on his drinking. The supervisor suggests, and Dr. Chou agrees, that it would be helpful to meet with Donald before the session to talk about both his father's drinking and the history of substance abuse in their family. Dr. Chou will encourage Donald to allow her to take the lead in talking with his father about his drinking.

The supervisor normalizes Dr. Chou's fear about meeting with this potentially volatile family. The supervisor advises Dr. Chou to provide structure for the family meeting, beginning with a good orientation, and gives her specific, practical scripts for setting limits with the monopolizer and the angry, out-of-control member. The supervisor reminds Dr. Chou that a "successful meeting" will be one in which she does her best to give the family the opportunity to come together and discuss their issues, and that she is not responsible for solving the family's problems. Despite the supervisor's reassurances and strategies for intervening, Dr. Chou remains anxious and concerned that the meeting will not go well. Supportively, the supervisor shares, "When I find myself in a difficult family meeting and I'm growing anxious and the meeting is spiraling out of control and despite my best efforts I can't get the meeting back on track, I stop and mentally say to myself, `What do I care if this family doesn't want to work together!'" Dr. Chou laughs. The supervisor allows, "Of course I care about the families I treat, and I would never say out loud anything so outrageous, yet this ridiculous little mental reminder helps me regain focus, composure, and objectivity." The supervisor reminds her that if the family meeting deteriorates despite her interventions, Dr. Chou should tell the family, "I think we need to take a short break so everyone can regroup and calm down. A short break may be helpful in getting us back on track." Dr. Chou should tell the family that she will leave the room for five minutes and will return and they will resume the meeting. Taking a short break often brings the out-of-control family up short and is an intervention that can dissipate mounting tension. A short break also helps Dr. Chou gather her thoughts about how best to proceed.

The Resident's Intervention

Dr. Chou begins the meeting by introducing her supervisor and explaining that she will be sitting in on the meeting. Dr. Chou then orients the family, asking each family member what he or she thinks is going to happen in today's meeting, and then feeds back each person's response. Dr. Chou tells the family that the meeting will last about one hour and that, in the interest of time, once she understands each of their concerns, she may have to interrupt discussions to move on, because they have a lot to cover and everyone has to have a chance to participate. Dr. Chou explains that she wants to make certain that at the end of the meeting they have a "blueprint," an understanding of the important family issues from everyone's perspective.

Donald's father, a large and powerful man, starts the meeting by saying that Donald is no longer going to hold the family hostage with his drinking and doing drugs, staying out all night, and cursing the family. He says, "I won't have my son be a drunk and a criminal." Immediately, Donald challenges his father saying, "You were a drunk for most of your life. We used to have to pull *you* out of bars! You're a (expletive) hypocrite and you're still drinking!" Mrs. Rizzo begins to cry as her husband counters and starts yelling at Donald, "I won't have you speak to me so disrespectfully!" Donald's sister is silent and sits with her head down. Dr. Chou empathically but firmly says, "I can see that tempers and feelings are pretty intense. We need to establish some ground rules for this meeting or we're not going to get anywhere." Donald rejoins, "I'm out of this (expletive) meeting," and stands up. Dr. Chou asks Donald to please sit down, which he does. Dr. Chou continues, "I understand that discussing these things is upsetting, but I can't allow cursing and arguing. If we are going to continue, one person will speak at a time and everyone needs to be respectful of one another. Does everyone agree? Do you want to go forward with this meeting?" The parents say that they want to continue the meeting. Dr. Chou asks Donald if he can abide by the rules, and Donald says yes. His sister nods in agreement.

Mr. Rizzo starts to talk about Donald's truancy, suspension from school, and appearance in court. Dr. Chou listens carefully and begins to feel anxious as she recognizes that the father is lecturing and monopolizing the session. Dr. Chou knows that she needs to set limits with him. She intervenes, thanking him for his summary of the issues and saying, "Remember, at the beginning of this meeting I said that I might have to interrupt when I understand what you are saying? I'm going to have to ask you to stop now and let us hear from others." Referring back to the orientation and reminding the family about asking members to stop talking is a respectful and nonshaming way of setting limits. The father stops talking. Dr. Chou asks the mother about her concerns. As Mrs. Rizzo begins to describe how upset and worried she is about Donald, the father starts talking, interrupting her. Donald's mother becomes silent. Dr. Chou listens for a while and then intervenes, telling the father, "I hear how concerned you are about Donald, but we really should have his mother finish sharing her concerns." The father apologizes for talking so much, and the mother starts again. When Dr. Chou asks Donald's sister if she has any concerns, she shakes her head no. Dr. Chou attempts to engage Lily by saying, "It might be hard to speak up in this meeting. Is it OK for me to check in with you as we go along?" Lily nods her head in the affirmative.

The father repeats that Donald must stop drinking and must abide by the rules of the house. Donald is very upset and says that his father always picks on him, saying to his father, "Yeah, what about your drinking?" Mr. Rizzo and Donald start arguing and escalate into a shouting match. Dr. Chou intervenes, asking the family, "Is this what happens at home?" Mrs. Rizzo says, "Yes, they argue all the time, and it's so upsetting." Dr. Chou asks Lily what she thinks. Lily replies, "My father and Donald are always yelling at each other." Dr. Chou asked her how she feels when that happens. She replies, "I get scared, but now I'm kind of used to it." At this point in the session, Dr. Chou says to the family, "Mr. Rizzo and Donald, you must stop arguing and yelling at each other or we won't accomplish anything in this meeting." Dr. Chou says, "Mr. Rizzo, you certainly are concerned about Donald's drinking and self-destructive behaviors, but it also sounds as though Donald worries about your drinking. If we are going to discuss these concerns, you both must be respectful and calm down." Dr. Chou turns to Donald, "I know you are trying to address your father's drinking, but when you verbally attack your father and start yelling, everyone becomes upset and focuses on your behavior rather than listening to your concerns. Do you understand that your yelling and cursing is getting in the way of people's listening to you and taking you seriously? Do you understand how you are coming across in this meeting? You want your family to consider your concerns, don't you?"

Donald takes a breath and quietly begins again. "My father says he quit drinking but I know he still does." Dr. Chou acknowledges that Donald is speaking respectfully about his concerns. Dr. Chou suggests that Donald ask his father directly about his drinking. Donald turns to his father and says in a quiet tone, "How come you're all over me and you do the same thing?"

Mr. Rizzo is silent for what seems like a long time, then finally admits that he does occasionally drink; then he talks about how drinking is a long-standing problem for him. He goes on to say, "I am concerned that Donald is going to ruin his future if he keeps drinking and doing drugs." Dr. Chou asks Donald what he thinks about what his father is saying. Donald replies, "Dad usually just yells at me. No one ever talks to Dad about his drinking." Dr. Chou asks the family what they think about what Donald is saying. Donald's mother initially is silent but finally agrees, "Maybe that's true." Encouraged by Dr. Chou, she goes on. "I am worried about my husband and about Donald. My husband drinks occasionally and I do get nervous that his drinking will increase. I know he shouldn't drink at all." Dr. Chou asks the parents if they talk about Mr. Rizzo's drinking. Mrs. Rizzo responds, "Yes, but not in front of the children." Dr. Chou asks the parents how it has felt to discuss the father's drinking in this family meeting. Mrs. Rizzo says, "I'm relieved. I just want Donald and his father to get along and both of them to stop drinking." Mr. Rizzo agrees that it is helpful to finally talk about things honestly. Dr. Chou checks in with Lily, who says that she knows that both Donald and her father drink too much. Dr. Chou says to the family, "While both Dad and Donald have been angry and arguing in this meeting, I see a family who care very much about one another and are concerned about both Dad's and Donald's drinking." Mrs. Rizzo says, "This is the first time we've been able to talk about problems as a family without ending up in a shouting match." Dr. Chou asks Donald's sister how she thinks the meeting is going. Does she have any concerns? Lily says she is worried about Donald. Dr. Chou replies, "Everyone seems to be worried about Donald." Lily continues, "Dad gets angry and yells at Donald a lot." She looks very sad. Dr. Chou asks her how she feels when her father gets angry and yells at Donald. She replies, "It's upsetting. I just want the yelling to stop." Dr. Chou addresses both Donald and his father, saying, "You can see how upsetting the arguing and yelling is for her." Dr. Chou asks if Donald and his father can agree to stop the arguing and yelling. They agree.

As the meeting comes to an end, Donald's mother asks him if he will stop smoking marijuana. Donald agrees that he will. His mother also expresses concern that abusing alcohol and marijuana will contribute to his suicidal thoughts, and Dr. Chou agrees. His mother suggests that AA would be good for both Donald and his father. Donald and his father agree that they will go together to AA meetings. The meeting ends with the family's feeling hopeful, and they state that the meeting has been productive. Dr. Chou realizes that she forgot to explore the issue of Donald's returning to school. She takes a few minutes while the family and Donald wait for discharge and inquires about school. Donald agrees to work on going back to school, and the parents seem pleased that Dr. Chou has taken the time to address the school issue.

Lessons Learned

The goals of the meeting have been met. This meeting was a success for the family in part because the father admitted to drinking and agreed to stop. If the father had continued to deny his drinking and to focus on Donald's drinking, at the very least Dr. Chou would have provided Donald and the family with a forum in which to safely confront the father.

The premeeting supervisory work anticipated the difficulties of the upcoming family meeting and helped Dr. Chou intervene effectively during the meeting. As a result of having the practical tools for setting limits, Dr. Chou was able to manage both her own anxiety and the family meeting.

SUMMARY

The resident who avoids the common mistakes can go on to successfully manage a difficult family meeting. Using role-playing and scripted responses can help residents learn to avoid these mistakes. It is particularly important to set limits for family members who act as the dominant powerbroker, the monopolizer,and the angry and challenging family, and for an out-of-control family. Good supervision includes role-playing and in situ observation.

CHAPTER SEVEN

Other Inpatient Interventions

Multifamily Psychoeducational Groups and Genograms

This chapter rounds out the skill mastery section by introducing two other family-oriented interventions — multifamily psychoeducational groups and the mapping of family patterns using a genogram — both of which can be easily adapted for the inpatient unit. Co-leading a multifamily psychoeducational group provides the resident another vehicle for learning to understand the concerns of family members and how to communicate empathetically with families. The use of a genogram facilitates talking with an individual patient or family about multigenerational family strengths and weaknesses and is helpful in individual and family assessment and therapy. Genogram groups are a way to work on family issues in a group format. An example of a genogram is provided.

MULTIFAMILY PSYCHOEDUCATIONAL GROUPS

Inpatient multifamily groups provide patients and family members with information about symptoms and the diagnosis of psychiatric illnesses, treatment options, and hospital and community resources. Providing psychoeducation to the families of patients has been shown to contribute to sustained clinical improvement for patients at discharge, especially for female patients and patients with chronic schizophrenia or bipolar disorder (Glick et al. 1993). As the APA Practice Guidelines indicate, families of patients with chronic mental illness should be offered family intervention, and this can begin on the inpatient unit (APA Work Groups 2000, 2002, 2004).

Establishing an inpatient multifamily group is relatively simple. All patients and their family members and friends are invited to the group, which meets at the end of visiting hours. The goals for the meeting are to introduce patients and their families to the multifamily group format, to provide psychoeducation, and to provide information on community resources. These groups are typically co-led by a resident and a clinical social worker or a psychiatric nurse, both of whom are knowledgeable about mental illness and community resources such as the National Alliance of the Mentally Ill (NAMI). Pamphlets from these organizations can be available at the meetings. Members of NAMI or other consumer groups can also be invited as guest speakers.

The leaders begin by explaining that family members may ask general questions about psychiatric illnesses, the mental health system, and available treatments, but that all specific questions about a relative's illness or treatment plan should be addressed to the patient's treatment team. The groups usually run from a half-hour to an hour, depending on the interest of those present. The focus is on encouraging families to provide mutual support, especially the sharing of strategies for coping with mental illness. Multifamily groups emphasize the importance of a support network to help family members. Group leaders answer general questions and guide the discussion toward topics such as the role of the family as advocate for the patient, the role of the family in treatment, how to deal with the stigma of mental illness, and how to access community support. Patients and family members often want to discuss ways to explain the patient's absence from the community. Leaders console families by reminding them that not all people need to be informed about the psychiatric hospitalization. Encouraging family members to discuss whom to tell and how to explain the hospitalization may be useful in reducing anxiety for patients as well as family members.

The group members can learn a great deal from each other. For example, patients and families who have been living with mental illness for years can be of great comfort to the newly diagnosed patient and family by offering strategies for coping with the illness and for working with the mental health system. Often the most helpful and effective feedback for a patient who is having a difficult time will come from another patient or family. A frustrated family member may learn more from a person outside his or her own family.

One common question posed in multifamily groups is how to get family members to understand that a mental illness is a medical condition, not a choice.

The establishment of more extensive family psychoeducational groups than the one described above requires a significant organizational commitment. Details of such programs are provided in Chapter 11.

The following discussion in a multifamily group illustrates how patients' and families' perspectives about the effects of the illness differ. Discussion of these differences between patients and family members fosters greater understanding and collaboration as they all live with mental illness.

CASE EXAMPLE:
A MULTIFAMILY PSYCHOEDUCATIONAL GROUP

Bob, a 30-year-old man with bipolar illness who is depressed, opens the group by sharing that he is upset over his wife's attempts to "micromanage" his life. He shares with the group that she "hovers over me constantly" and "I can't have a bad day! My wife constantly checks up on me!" Mary, a 42-year-old woman who is recovering from a manic episode, rejoins, "If I'm having a good time, am happy or silly, my family overacts and thinks I'm getting manic!" Other patients in the group echo these concerns, with statements like, "Family members need to understand that we know best how to conduct our lives. It's not helpful to treat us like children."

Josephine, a 35-year-old woman with depression, states, "Unless you have the illness, there is no way you can possibly understand what it's like." The group co-leader asks family members to respond. Several family members respond empathetically, "It's true, we can't possibly know what you're going through," "It breaks my heart to see my son ravaged by mania," and "My daughter tries so hard, but her unrelenting depression robbed her of her dream of becoming a lawyer, and I worry about her future." Family members also emphasize how devastating mental illness is for the family and that patients have little understanding of how mental illness affects the family. Nancy, the sister of Carolyn, who is 30 years of age and has bipolar illness, states, "I don't think my sister really understands how hard we try to help her. She stops taking her meds and becomes nasty, saying horrible things to our parents." John, father of Paul, a 28-year-old man with bipolar disorder, now manic, confesses, "I'm terrified that Paul will end up killing himself or someone else. Paul has been in an escalating manic state for weeks and he refused to call his psychiatrist. Thank God, the police took Paul to the hospital after they arrested him for driving over 100 miles an hour down Route 195 at 2 o'clock in the morning. They could just as easily have thrown him in jail. The officer told the hospital Paul was laughing, screaming, and totally out of control when they pulled him over. The officer said that his brother has bipolar illness, so he understood that Paul desperately needed help. But what about next time?" Diane, the wife of Jared, a 40-year-old physician who has depression, confides, "I fear that Jared will become so despondent that he'll kill himself. He's tried before. When Jared is depressed, I feel totally helpless, and I admit there are times I feel like screaming, 'Quit feeling so sorry for yourself. Do something; don't just lie there. You have a wife and daughter who need you.'" Diane continues, "I know when people are depressed they can't just pull themselves up by the bootstraps. In a way, Jared's depression has taken over all of our lives."

At this point the social worker asks how the group feels right now. Group members answer, "angry," "tense," and "upset." The co-leader shares his observation, "I can feel the tension and upset in the room but what's also evident is that everyone in this group has suffered as a result of mental illness. Is there a middle ground where patients and family members can work together to manage the illness?" The tension and upset in the room dissipates. The group members, with the help of the leader, begin to explore the need to compromise; patients are encouraged to be more responsible for staying in treatment and taking their medication, and family members are encouraged to respect the patient as an adult whose responsibility it is to manage his or her own illness.

The group leaders strongly suggest that each patient and his or her family develop a safety net, a plan for appropriate intervention when the patient begins to have difficulty, so the family can be there when needed by the patient but not intrude on the patient's independence. Such a plan would be designed by the patient, the family, and a member of the treatment team and might consist of (1) identifying early warning signs and symptoms; (2) establishing an agreement that the family will observe the patient for a day or two and, if symptoms continue to worsen, intervene by encouraging the patient to contact his or her psychiatrist; and (3) agreeing that the patient will be the one to contact the psychiatrist. The group members agree that such a safety plan would be helpful.

These sorts of exchanges are typical of multifamily psychoeducational groups, and they reflect how important the format can be for patients, family members, and clinicians (Keitner et al. 2002). Residents learn how to listen, summarize, and give feedback to the group members. The social worker demonstrates how to move the group forward to work on solutions that are appropriate for most members. And the resident is able to observe his or her patients in a social milieu and develop an appreciation of their interpersonal skills and progress during the hospitalization.

GENOGRAMS

A genogram is a family diagram that maps relationships and patterns of functioning across generations. Genograms have been used for years in therapy with families, and there is an extensive literature on their use (McGoldrick 2005). A genogram is a simple tool that provides an easy visual aid for the physician and the patient. It captures the multigenerational transmission of family patterns, which can help the patient and family develop a greater awareness of the influence of family factors on the illness (Bowen 1978). Additionally, the placement of a family genogram in the patient's chart provides all the involved clinicians with an easily accessible map of the key family members in a patient's life. Genograms can be tailored to work with almost any person or family, whatever the psychiatric diagnosis.

After the initial psychiatric interview with the patient, the resident will meet with the patient to review pertinent facts. If there are significant family issues, the resident and patient can construct a genogram mapping three generations. It is important to include relatives that are meaningful to the patient, who may be distant family or divorced or stepfamily members. The defining characteristics of each family member are written beside that member's name. When themes emerge, they can be written on the genogram (e.g., "Our family demonstrates care for one another by becoming overly involved and anxious about each other"). The resident should draw the patient's attention to patterns and continually invite the patient to formulate his own analysis of the meaning behind the patterns. As emotional legacies can be both positive and negative, the resident will encourage the patient to formulate one list of family attributes the patient would like to develop and another of those family attributes the patient would like to minimize. By tracking intergenerational patterns, patients can alter their understanding of various family members and of themselves. For example, the offspring of divorced parents have the opportunity to talk equally and nonjudgmentally about each parent.

In families with young children, play genograms may be used: A family outline is mapped on a large board. The child is invited to choose from a group of specific toy objects those items that they identify with family members. The items are then placed on the family map (McGoldrick 2005). The child is encouraged to explain the object choices depicting family members. These play genograms can be used with whole families and may encourage dialogue in families who are guarded or reluctant to discuss family issues.

Genograms can also be completed by patients simultaneously in a group format. The patients must be able to concentrate for the duration of the task and be able to tolerate some exploration of family issues. Ideally, there will be two to six participants, and the session will last an hour. At the beginning of a group genogram session, the therapist carefully explains ground rules, such as the need for patient confidentiality and the need to respect self-disclosure; the group will use only first names, and all agree not to discuss outside the session what is talked about within the group. The goal of the session may be explained in the following way: "Often we go through our days unaware that we are dealing with life in a similar way to our preceding relatives. We cope as they coped. By identifying patterns of learned behaviors, we become free to alter the way in which we react and behave. One way to illustrate these patterns is through the use of a genogram. Participants will draw their family tree and map important relationships and influences. If anyone anticipates becoming distressed or does not wish to contribute, he or she can refrain."

The group leader illustrates how to construct a genogram by drawing a hypothetical genogram on a board in front of the group, showing how family patterns are passed down from generation to generation, almost like a favorite food recipe. (In Rhode Island, many participants talk about the recipe for tomato sauce that has been handed down through the generations!) The leader points out that some inherited coping styles are helpful and some may be problematic. Both types of patterns should be illustrated on the sample genogram. Questions about complicated family structural features, such as multiple marriages, are answered. Participants then draw their own family genograms, mapping three generations of members and adding descriptive adjectives beside each member whom the participants know well enough to describe. Participants are encouraged to include positive attributes, with the purpose of highlighting strengths. These might include intelligence, kindness, wisdom, and competence. When patterns are noticed, such as alcohol use, mental illness, and over- or underinvolvement by members, these are discussed. The therapist asks how these attributes or beliefs have been passed down and how they affect the participant.

When most participants have completed their genograms, they are invited to share any discovered patterns. All members of the group are encouraged to participate in discussing what other persons' genograms reveal as well as their own. Before concluding the meeting, the leader should assess the stability of patients who participated in the project, as exploring family history can occasionally be disturbing. Group cohesion and calmness is maintained by facilitating a discussion that focuses on topics of low emotional intensity.

CASE EXAMPLE:
MR. PEREZ AND HIS ANGRY WIFE

Mr. Perez was admitted with depressive symptoms, alcohol intoxication, and cocaine abuse. He used money allocated for domestic bills to buy cocaine. The misappropriation of funds angered his wife. His substance abuse has affected the amount of time that he spends at home, further straining the marriage. When the resident called to arrange a family meeting, Ms. Perez emphatically stated that her husband had repeatedly lied to her and that she could no longer deal with his problems, but she agreed to come to a family meeting the next morning. That afternoon, the resident and Mr. Perez developed a genogram. Analysis of the family history exposed a long line of alcoholic and substance-abusing males in his family, as well as emotional and physical abuse perpetrated by his father. (Figure 7.1 portrays the genogram developed with Mr. Perez.) Mr. Perez described the difficult and traumatic relationship he had with his father and regretted that they had not been able to resolve their differences before his father died. Mr. Perez

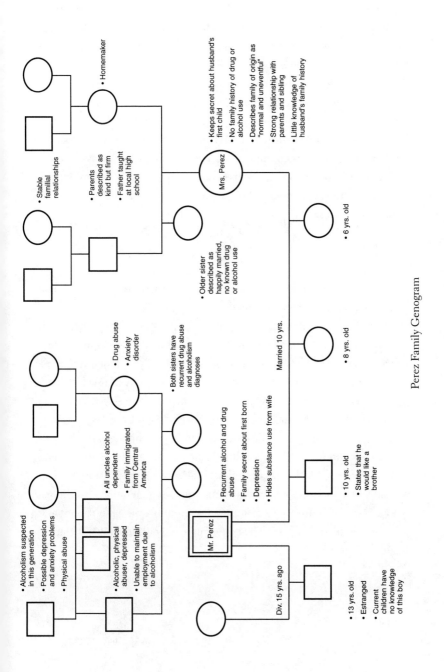

Perez Family Genogram

- Alcoholism suspected in this generation
- Possible depression and anxiety problems
- Physical abuse

- All uncles alcohol dependent
- Family immigrated from Central America

- Alcoholic, physical abuser, depressed
- Unable to maintain employment due to alcoholism

- Stable familial relationships

- Parents described as kind but firm
- Father taught at local high school

- Drug abuse
- Anxiety disorder

- Both sisters have recurrent drug abuse and alcoholism diagnoses

- Older sister described as happily married, no known drug or alcohol use

- Keeps secret about husband's first child
- No family history of drug or alcohol use
- Describes family of origin as "normal and uneventful"
- Strong relationship with parents and sibling
- Little knowledge of husband's family history

Mr. Perez

- Recurrent alcohol and drug abuse
- Family secret about first born
- Depression
- Hides substance use from wife

Mrs. Perez

Married 10 yrs.

Div. 15 yrs. ago

- 13 yrs. old
- Estranged
- Current children have no knowledge of this boy

- 10 yrs. old
- States that he would like a brother

- 8 yrs. old

- 6 yrs. old

shared his genogram with his wife when she came to visit him that evening. At the beginning of the family meeting the next morning, Ms. Perez exclaimed with great excitement that she now understood the extent of her husband's problem. She was astonished to see so many alcoholics in his family and to learn that her husband had grown up in a violent alcoholic household. She immediately comprehended the implications of this history for her husband, and she committed herself to helping him defy his family legacy of alcoholism and drug abuse. The remainder of the meeting focused on examining the poor communication and problem-solving skills in the family and on devising ways for Mr. Perez to improve his relationship with his son. With his wife involved in his treatment, Mr. Perez has a greatly improved prognosis.

SUMMARY

Residents can participate in conducting inpatient psychoeducational groups for patients and their families. Co-leading such groups gives them the opportunity to observe their patients in a group setting, which often leads to a greater understanding of their strengths and weaknesses. The resident will also learn how to respond to questions from family members of varying sophistication and to use the group process for a variety of psychoeducational goals. This training will prove invaluable for the resident in leading community-based educational seminars after graduation.

Using genograms with individual patients can enhance care, through the identification of family and cultural patterns that influence the patient. As in the case of Mr. Perez, an understanding of a family history of alcoholism and associated behaviors throughout past generations can help a patient and the family move forward, away from blaming the patient and to an active treatment plan. The genogram can be adapted to a variety of treatment settings.

PART FOUR

Challenges in Working with Families

CHAPTER EIGHT

The Resident's Perspective

Attitudes and Fears

Meeting with families can be intimidating for residents. Residents who are anxious may avoid meeting with families, making excuses—there's no time, or it isn't their job. The role of the supervising physician is to model how to handle uncertainty in diagnosis or management in the family meeting and to help residents be self-reflective regarding their own clinical strengths and weaknesses. A case example describes a resident who is anxious about being seen as incompetent by the patient and the family. The supervisor provides strategies for managing the family meeting.

Family work can be intimidating for the psychiatry resident, who typically feels anxious and uncertain when meeting with the families of inpatients. While the literature on working with families is rich in theory, it gives little attention to practitioners' worries as they begin to work with families. These concerns need to be actively addressed in supervision, or the resident may resist working with families, to the detriment of the patient.

"IT'S NOT MY JOB TO MEET WITH FAMILIES; I WORK WITH PATIENTS."

On the typical inpatient psychiatry service, the primary focus for the psychiatric resident is on developing skills in interviewing individual patients, becoming proficient in diagnosis, establishing a treatment plan, and prescribing psychiatric medications. When the attending psychiatrist values family involvement and is skilled in meeting with families, residents tend also to embrace family work. Alternatively, if the attending psychiatrist has little interaction with the families of the inpatients, there will be no clear expectation that the resident meet with families. Attending psychiatrists who are biologically trained may not see the relevance of including families in an inpatient's assessment and treatment.

The importance of the supervising physician as a professional role model cannot be underestimated. There is nothing more powerful than seeing your supervisor admit to a family that he or she does not know what is wrong with their family member but will work hard to find out and to help the patient. It is difficult for physicians, especially residents, to acknowledge that they do not know the diagnosis and therefore cannot determine the best treatment plan. They mistakenly believe that they must put on an expert face in all situations. Residents see themselves as unskilled and may believe that it takes extensive training to be able to work effectively with families. Thus, good role modeling can show residents how to accept the limitations of their knowledge and how to interact empathetically with families.

"I DON'T HAVE TIME TO MEET WITH FAMILIES."

Residents often say that they don't have time to meet with families. This statement usually masks the resident's feelings of insecurity and uncertainty about how to interact with families, and it can be a way of avoiding the "angry" or "demanding" family. It should be acknowledged that a family in a crisis can be difficult to tolerate. In an attempt to manage his or her own anxiety, the resident may attach labels to the family members, especially the most outspoken member, and make pejorative statements to the other team members, such as, "That mother's a borderline!" As residents learn about families and become more aware of the family's perspective, they develop more empathy toward the family. (Chapter 9 describes the perspective of the family in detail.) Reframing is a useful technique for managing one's attitude toward "difficult" families, and it can lead to a powerful intervention. The resident can say to him- or herself that the "difficult" family members are "educated consumers who are advocating for their rel-

ative." The resident can then say to the family, "You are right, you are trying your best to help your relative. He is lucky to have you advocating for
him. If I were in your shoes, I would be doing the same thing." The resident thus supports and praises the family members and makes a helpful
correction in his or her own perspective. Following up with the promise,
"We will do our best to get those answers for you" reassures the family and
reminds the resident that mental illness affects not only the patient but the
family. Families respond, in our experience, very positively to this honest
and affirming approach.

"I'M ANXIOUS AND FEARFUL ABOUT MEETING WITH THE FAMILY."

From the resident's perspective, meeting with a family can seem a daunting task, because the resident must "take leadership, condensing the mass of
clinical options into a practical, sensible, well organized interview with a
group of strangers" (Weber, McKeever, and McDaniel 1985, p. 357). Residents are unlikely to talk openly about their anxieties and fears, instead
becoming avoidant, showing up late, or being unprepared. Physicians are
socialized in the medical profession to be problem solvers; they are expected
to have all the answers and to be able to identify and fix the problems. Physicians are expected to be the authority who never shows anxiety or uncertainty. Medicine has been described as glorifying machismo, with the effect
of turning both male and female medical students into macho doctors who
have all the answers (Klass 1987). Training in medical school has been
likened to boot camp, and if you don't fit the mold, then you don't belong.
Thus, residents hesitate to meet with families if they don't have a definitive
diagnosis or treatment plan, fearing that the family will perceive them as
inept. Residents do not easily acknowledge or discuss perceived imperfec-
tions, such as being anxious. Discussion of anxieties and fears should therefore be facilitated as soon as possible and normalized, as it is unlikely that
residents will address these concerns without prompting. When these difficulties are made explicit, the resident can see his or her struggle as part of
the normal process of professional development. Self-reflection and exploration of personal strengths and weaknesses need to be acknowledged as
important parts of the learning process.

"I'M OVERWHELMED AND OUTNUMBERED AND I DON'T KNOW WHAT TO DO."

Residents are often reluctant to meet with families because family work is labor intensive and the dynamic possibilities within the family are endless. If asked, many residents admit that during a family meeting, they feel outnumbered, have difficulty tolerating the movement and flow of dialogue, and often feel overwhelmed. They must manage the family meeting, giving each family member time to express concerns, and then make sense of it all by the end of the meeting. Residents report not knowing what to do with all of the issues families identify as problematic. Many residents ask, "How do I incorporate the multiple perspectives of the family into a meaningful session? Which issues do I explore in depth? If I explore a 'hot' issue, what do I do if the family starts arguing? Do I stop them from arguing and try to refocus the meeting? What if that doesn't work? How do I get them back on track?" These are all important questions that are addressed in this book. Residents can be reassured that, with practice, they will master these skills.

"WHAT IF THE FAMILY MEETING GETS OUT OF CONTROL?"

Residents are often fearful that they will become the target of the family's hostility and that the family meeting will get out of control. Anxious and distraught families often have difficulty managing their feelings while trying to understand what is happening to their hospitalized relative. Sometimes a family member will become angry and may be verbally aggressive, questioning the resident's competence. The hostile family can be difficult for the most seasoned professional to handle, but for the resident it can be a nightmare. While it is important to attempt to engage the hostile family as an ally and part of the treatment team, practical strategies for countering verbal assaults and techniques for ending the meeting must become part of the resident's repertoire. When the family is so upset or hostile toward the resident that the session is no longer productive, the resident must be able to end the meeting. The resident must firmly state to the family that while he or she understands how upsetting the session has been, attacking people is not helpful, and unless it stops, the meeting is over. The resident can tell the family that they can meet again, if and when they are able to participate constructively.

Residents' anxieties are lessened if they use structure to effectively handle the myriad of family situations that arise in a session. Bringing structure to the family interview reduces the resident's feelings of being out of control and assists the resident in minimizing the family's dynamic interactions. Such structured assessment tools are the Global Assessment of Relational Functioning (APA 2000) and the McMaster Model of Family Functioning (Ryan et al. 2005). Case examples illustrating the use of these assessment tools are found in Chapter 5.

"IT'S NOT PSYCHIATRY, IT'S REAL LIFE!"

Working with families moves the trainee away from psychiatry into real-life experience, in which the trainee might feel less confident. Residents are often recently married or in the "honeymoon stage" of their own family development and may avoid dealing with families in difficulty to help preserve the myth of "happily ever after." Residents express feelings of discomfort in delving into "family issues," and families are reluctant to talk about intimacy problems and family secrets. A resident may be uncomfortable discussing sexuality with couples who are their parents' or grandparents' age. It is important for residents to overcome their reluctance to ask about difficult family issues, as these problems can have significant effects on the patients' well-being and because patients and families themselves are unlikely to bring them up, perceiving them as irrelevant to the physician, who they think wants to know about only symptoms and medication effects.

CASE EXAMPLE: THE LONG-SUFFERING PARENTS AND THE GIFTED SON

The case of Brandon illustrates how a supervisor and resident might discuss the resident's anxiety, practical suggestions for handling difficult situations, and the structure of an inpatient family meeting.

Brandon is a 22-year-old man with a diagnosis of schizoaffective disorder. He has been admitted after being found wandering the streets of Boston, believing he was a disciple of Buddha; he was walking to cure mankind of cruelty. Brandon was a brilliant 18-year-old sophomore at Brown University when he experienced his first psychotic break and spent several months in hospital. For psychiatric follow-up, he was sent to an exclusive wilderness psychiatric retreat in California, but he left after one month, refusing to follow the rules or take any medications. Brandon has had several hospitalizations since that time for delusional and grandiose thinking and has continued to smoke marijuana daily. He has seen outpatient psychiatrists but each time stopped treatment and dismissed the doctors as "incompetent." He has taken various antipsychotic medications, most recently ziprazodone, but he stopped that medication two months before the current admission to the hospital.

Brandon's parents are extremely supportive, both emotionally and economically. On several occasions, they arranged for Brandon to live independently in various apartments, but Brandon invariably got into arguments with other tenants because he played loud music at all hours and left trash everywhere. Before this admission, Brandon was living at home, where his behaviors were becoming increasingly out of control and threatening. He stayed in his room for hours reading Eastern philosophy and refused to bathe or come out for meals. He escalated from screaming at his father to pushing him up against a wall. He was verbally abusive toward his mother and would routinely lock his 10-year-old sister out of the house when his parents were at work.

Brandon hasn't eaten in three days; he says he is fasting to cleanse his spirit. Arriving on the adult inpatient unit, he refuses all medications and is arrogant and sarcastic with other patients. When his parents check on him after he is in place on the unit, Brandon is cool and demanding with his mother and openly sarcastic toward his father. On more than one occasion, the nurses observe Brandon being hostile toward his father. When meeting with the resident, Brandon tries to debate the validity of various psychoanalytic theories. Brandon tells the attending psychiatrist that he doesn't care to work with the resident, who is obviously a "neophyte," and that his own IQ is considerably higher than the resident's IQ.

The Resident's Concerns

Dr. Jones, a second-year resident, feels intimidated by Brandon. He tries to establish a working alliance with Brandon but Brandon, although sometimes pleasant, is often dismissive and disrespectful. During individual sessions, Brandon launches into long diatribes about philosophy and attempts to bait the resident into arguments. A family meeting has been scheduled for two days after admission. As the time of the meeting approaches, Dr. Jones tells his supervisor his fears about managing what is certain to be a volatile meeting with Brandon and his parents. What if Brandon starts verbally attacking his father or, worse, goes after his father physically? Dr. Jones has similar concerns about his own safety. What if it becomes obvious to the parents that Dr. Jones is anxious and uncertain as to how to handle the meeting? Will they ask that Brandon be seen by someone else? Brandon's father is a prominent physician, and this puts additional pressure on Dr. Jones. What is the point of the meeting if Brandon is going to refuse medications and insist on dictating treatment? What if Dr. Jones mismanages the meeting and is seen as incompetent?

The Supervisor's Response

The first important task of the supervisor is to clarify the purpose of the family meeting. From Brandon's perspective, meeting with his parents is unnecessary. Dr. Jones and Brandon's parents share the goal of helping Brandon agree to take medication so that he will stabilize and can return home. The supervisor agrees with the goal for the meeting. In addition, the supervisor expects that the parents will want to meet with the treatment team to learn how they can help Brandon's recovery.

The supervisor listens to Dr. Jones's concerns, then acknowledges and normalizes his anxieties and fears. As a result of the supervisor's empathetic and helpful stance, Dr. Jones feels less anxious and is able to focus on the practical strategies offered by the supervisor. The supervisor helps Dr. Jones outline a structured format for the meeting, reminding him that the purpose of the meeting is to help Brandon agree to take medication so that he will stabilize and be able to return home. The supervisor acknowledges that the meeting may well end up in a hostile confrontation between Brandon and his father. It is therefore imperative that Dr. Jones understand what he is and isn't responsible for regarding the family meeting. The supervisor works with the resident to accept that, while he will make his best effort to help Brandon and his parents, whether they work together is up to them. While Dr. Jones is responsible for providing an opportunity for them to discuss their problems, he is not responsible for resolving their issues for them.

Dr. Jones very much wants to help Brandon stay in control of his behavior if he starts to escalate during the session. The supervisor gives the resident specific examples of what to say to Brandon if he begins to yell and lose control: "Brandon, cursing or yelling at your father is not allowed in this meeting. I know it is difficult for you to meet with your father, but you must stay in control. What you have to say is important, but your screaming gets in the way of our being able to consider the points you're trying to make."

The supervisor demonstrates how to end the meeting if Brandon loses control. "Brandon, you're very upset and angry, and I've asked you to calm down, which you haven't been able to do. At this point we aren't making any progress and the meeting, in fact, is deteriorating, so I'm going to stop the meeting. Brandon, when you are able to calm down and participate appropriately, we can meet again." The supervisor recommends giving Brandon several chances to gain control and participate appropriately, but says that if those attempts fail, Dr. Jones should end the meeting. The supervisor will attend the meeting but intervene only at Dr. Jones's request or if the supervisor perceives that Dr. Jones needs assistance.

The Resident's Intervention

As the family meeting begins, sure enough, Brandon immediately attempts to take over. After a little while, Dr. Jones stops Brandon, saying, "I'm going to ask you to stop there, Brandon. We have about an hour to meet today and I want to make certain that everyone has a chance to share his or her concerns. We need to discuss what happened before your hospitalization, how your treatment is progressing, and a discharge plan." Brandon ignores Dr. Jones and continues talking. Dr. Jones firmly repeats that Brandon must stop and give others a chance to talk. Brandon becomes quiet. His father and mother talk about Brandon's dangerous and hostile behaviors. Brandon interrupts throughout but each time quiets down when Dr. Jones insists that he give his parents time to talk. As the meeting progresses, Brandon begins to raise his voice and curse at his father. Dr. Jones chooses not to address Brandon at this point. The parents continue and Brandon starts to escalate, yelling at his father. Dr. Jones tells Brandon that cursing and yelling will not be tolerated. Brandon curses at Dr. Jones. At this point Dr. Jones empathetically but firmly tells Brandon that, while he knows this meeting is difficult, Brandon must be respectful or he will have to return to the unit. Brandon settles down temporarily.

The parents tell Brandon that they want him to live with them after discharge from the hospital and are willing to work with him to go back to school (a goal that Brandon had identified) but that he must take medication while in the hospital and as an outpatient. Brandon protests, saying that he will decide what is best for himself. Dr. Jones asks Brandon if he will consider taking medication, a condition of his parents' allowing him to return home and work toward getting back to college. Brandon stands up and announces, "This meeting is over" and walks out of the room. Dr. Jones continues to talk with the parents, who are disappointed but not surprised at Brandon's response. The parents share that this hostile and disrespectful behavior is what they have been living with for years. They describe how despondent they are and how ineffective they feel. Brandon's mother expresses guilt, saying, "I feel that we've failed Brandon in some way. I chose to go back to work when Brandon was 11 years old. Maybe if I had stayed home or we had been stricter with him things would be different." Dr. Jones takes this opportunity to reach out to Brandon's parents. He says, "Unfortunately, parents often feel overly responsible for their children's behavior." Dr. Jones and the parents discuss Brandon's diagnosis of schizoaffective disorder. While the parents are knowledgeable about their son's mental illness, they continue to feel guilt and remorse. Dr. Jones reassures them, saying that he can see how concerned they are and how devoted to their son they are. He explains that he will work with Brandon, hoping to help him gain better control over his behaviors, and will encourage him to participate in another family meeting. Dr. Jones and the parents discuss their fears that even if Brandon is medication compliant in the hospital he may choose to discontinue his medicine after discharge.

Over the course of the next two weeks, Brandon is calmer on the unit, less argumentative and less grandiose with the staff. He has responded well to both the structure of the unit and his daily sessions with Dr. Jones. Finally, Brandon and his parents are able to have a more successful family meeting. The parents continue to insist on Brandon's taking medication before he is allowed to come home. Brandon behaves more appropriately in the second meeting and does not curse when he disagrees with his parents. He reluctantly agrees to take medication and is started on risperidone. He verbalizes that he understands that he must take his medication to be able to return to live with his parents.

Lessons Learned

The goal of the family meetings is met—Brandon agrees to take his medication in order to return to live with his parents. Also, Brandon is able to participate appropriately in the second family meeting and articulates that he needs to take medication to aid in his recovery. Dr. Jones survives the meetings and develops valuable skills in managing his own anxiety and fear in dealing with a volatile patient. He learns that, while being empathetic and firm and setting appropriate limits does not guarantee a successful outcome of a family meeting, he did succeed in containing the patient's affect and his own anxiety and providing support to the parents. He modeled to the parents how to remain calm and detached while keeping to basic issues, and he demonstrated how to avoid lecturing to or debating with Brandon. The resident thus supports the parents' efforts in setting limits with Brandon. Although Brandon stormed out of the first session, in the subsequent meeting he and his parents were able to move toward problem resolution. Dr. Jones learned that while he can provide the opportunity to address problems and guidance on working toward their resolution, the family members are ultimately responsible for the functioning of their family. Remembering that the family style of interaction had been long established helps Dr. Jones be realistic in assessing what can be accomplished during Brandon's hospital stay.

SUMMARY

The resident who has the skills needed to manage a family meeting can provide optimal patient care. The supervisor guides the resident by acknowledging his or her fears and anxieties and laying the groundwork for the resident to learn further skills in working with families. The supervisor must review the resident's concerns in supervisory sessions before and after the family meeting. Failure to address the resident's anxieties and fears will result in the resident's continued avoidance of meeting with families.

CHAPTER NINE

The Family's Perspective

Sources of Anxiety

This chapter outlines the fears and anxieties that family members often experience when they attend a meeting with a psychiatrist. Family members typically fear that they will be blamed for the patient's problems, and they may already believe that they have failed; this is especially true of mothers of hospitalized children or young adults. Children, especially children of divorced parents, are also hesitant to speak up, for fear that they will get in trouble with their parents. It is extremely helpful to the resident in managing his or her own anxiety to appreciate how difficult it can be for family members to participate in a family meeting. A case example is described in which the patient and his divorced parents are hesitant to meet as a family. Supervisor-resident discussion prior to and after the family meeting is outlined. Family skills supervision helps the resident by providing strategies for both acknowledging and managing the anxieties and fears of each family member.

Historically, psychiatry has been organized around an individual-treatment paradigm with a legacy of exclusion of families. Residents usually adopt the assumptions about families that prevail within the profession, and they may therefore, unfortunately, develop negative prejudices about families. They may anticipate hostility and resistance when meeting with families. But if residents have qualms about meeting with the family, families are typically more anxious than the professionals at the prospect of having a family meeting. Some members of most families, and all members of some families, are reluctant to attend a family meeting.

Family members confronting the mental health system fear being blamed for the patient's problems. Parents of offspring with psychiatric problems usually have internalized society's view that the parents, especially the mother, are at least partially to blame for the aberrant behavior. And yet, by their very presence at a family meeting, parents are acknowledging that they have been unsuccessful in resolving family conflicts, and they likely feel a sense of failure. In addition, they may be frightened for their ill family member, frustrated at the failure of their attempts to help, and still holding out hope that maybe this time something will work. For intact families, a family meeting can be complicated and daunting, but if the parents are divorced or if stepparents and stepchildren are involved, the family faces an even greater challenge in meeting together. Tension is likely to be high, and conflicts in loyalty, especially for the children, can be a major issue. In any family meeting, children may fear that if they speak up, they will get into trouble or they will get their parents into trouble. Children, too, may be carrying around a belief that the problems are their fault. During the meeting, family members typically feel stressed as they anticipate being criticized and confronted when problems and conflicts are explored. They feel put on the spot when asked to comment on other members' perspectives and perhaps to compromise their position, even as they struggle to manage their own emotions during discussions of family problems. And family members often feel intimidated by the elements of the mental health system—the doctors, the specialized language, not to mention the complexities of hospital admission.

While family meetings can be beneficial therapeutically, they are stressful for all family members, including the patient. Individual psychotherapy focuses on mirroring, empathy, and acceptance for the individual, who also receives the undivided attention of the psychiatrist or therapist for fifty minutes. However, in family meetings, patients and family members must share the attention and time of the psychiatrist, must tolerate listening to the concerns of others, and will probably be confronted and asked to make changes. The resident should prepare the inpatient for how the upcoming family meeting will differ from individual psychotherapy: that each family member will have an equal chance to state concerns, that everyone will have to listen respectfully to others. The resident can anticipate with the patient that the meeting may be uncomfortable. They can explore any questions the patient may have about the upcoming meeting and talk about what the patient thinks the family will be sharing. The resident can reassure the patient that what they have discussed in individual therapy will remain confidential. Having this discussion before the family session both reassures the patient and makes him or her better able to participate in the meeting.

CASE EXAMPLE: MARK AND HIS DIVORCED, BICKERING PARENTS

Mark, a 16-year-old high school sophomore living with his mother, was hospitalized with major depression. He is an only child, and his parents have been divorced for 12 years. His mother has bipolar disorder but is stable and works part-time at a flower shop. His father, a college professor, had had monthly visits with his son but has recently pulled away from him. Mark is an outstanding athlete and, until recently, was an honor student at a local private high school. According to Mark, the events leading up to the admission include: (1) his father recently informed Mark that he would no longer pay child support and told Mark to tell his mother; (2) his father had canceled the last few monthly visits with Mark; (3) his mother has been increasingly upset regarding the loss of child support and asked Mark to intervene with his father; (4) Mark is very upset about constantly being put in the middle between his bickering parents; and (5) Mark fears that if he confronts his father, his father will become angry and they will have even less contact than they do now.

Dr. Chandler, a second-year resident, initially meets with Mark and his mother. They spend the majority of the meeting talking about their concerns regarding Mark's father. Dr. Chandler contacts Mark's father to arrange for a meeting. The father indicates that he is going out of town soon but can come for one meeting. Dr. Chandler would have preferred to meet with Mark and his father, as he did with Mark and his mother, and then have a follow-up meeting with both parents and Mark. Instead, because Mark's father can come for only one meeting, Dr. Chandler agrees to go straight to a meeting with both parents and Mark.

The Resident's Concerns

In discussing the upcoming family meeting in supervision, Dr. Chandler mentions being aware of how difficult it is going to be for Mark's divorced parents to deal with each other in the meeting. Dr. Chandler is concerned that Mark's father might believe that he will be blamed and be put on the hot seat during the meeting, because Mark had told his father how upset his mother is about losing the child support. Also, Mark's father may feel that he is at a disadvantage, as Dr. Chandler has already met with Mark's mother and heard her side of the story. He realizes that some strategic planning is needed to be sure that everyone's concerns are addressed without a full-scale argument breaking out. Dr. Chandler is concerned that this meeting might make things worse for Mark.

The Supervisor's Response

The supervisor begins by clarifying the purpose of the family meeting. Mark wants the meeting with his father. Dr. Chandler wants to meet with the parents to help them understand how their continued bickering and putting Mark in the middle is contributing to Mark's depression. Also, the supervisor points out, the meeting can be useful for establishing ground rules for how the parents will interact with Mark in the future. The supervisor acknowledges Dr. Chandler's anxiety about the upcoming meeting and asks Dr. Chandler to think about what Mark's parents are feeling about the meeting. Dr. Chandler says that they must be dreading getting together and that Mark and his parents are probably more worried about the meeting than he is.

Dr. Chandler asks for suggestions on how to facilitate a discussion of the parents' pattern of communicating and arguing with each other through Mark. How can he help these parents? The supervisor recommends, first, that Dr. Chandler establish an alliance with each family member. The supervisor advises the resident to begin the session by welcoming Mark's parents and acknowledging that it is both important and difficult for them to be there. The supervisor recommends normalizing the parents' dilemma by saying that although it is difficult for divorced parents to meet, it is important for children of divorced parents to have both parents involved.

Dr. Chandler should begin the session with Mark's father, because he has not yet had an opportunity to talk. This might help to neutralize any feeling of bias that the father might have, knowing that there has already been a meeting with Mark and his mother. Dr. Chandler is to listen carefully to Mark's father, give him feedback to assure him that his perspective has been understood, and then have Mark's mother articulate her concerns. Dr. Chandler is to give feedback to the mother about her concerns and then move on to Mark. The supervisor emphasizes the importance of not allowing people to interrupt or challenge each other on what's being said. Dr. Chandler is to remind the family that he needs to hear each person's perspective on the issues and that everyone will have a chance to speak.

Dr. Chandler is cautioned by his supervisor not to allow the family to launch into a lengthy debate or disagreement over the issues during this first session. If this begins to happen, Dr. Chandler needs to intervene quickly and say, "At this point I am trying to gather basic information about the problems you face as a family, and while I know this is difficult, we really do need to speak one at a time and not interrupt. I will make certain that each of you gets to tell your side of the story." Another helpful intervention is to say to family members who are arguing and disagreeing on an issue, "Is this what happens when you try to discuss this issue at home?" The family usually says yes, and the resident can follow that up with, "I can see that you have very different opinions on this issue, so at this point I must ask you to agree to disagree." This intervention acknowledges the family's differences and allows the session to move forward. Dr. Chandler also should prevent the family from diverting the meeting from its main purpose. In addition, allowing the parents to argue reestablishes their respective positions and results in entrenchment and erosion of the goals for the family meeting. Dr. Chandler must help the family understand that the goals of the meeting are to begin talking about the problems and listening to each other and to come to an agreement on how best to help Mark.

The Resident's Intervention

The night before the family meeting, Dr. Chandler finds Mark crying inconsolably. Through tears of anger and grief Mark shares how his childhood has been one of trying to be the perfect son and trying to manage his parents' hatred of each other. Mark asks how, even if his father agrees to pay for college, he can leave his mother; he fears she will become ill again. Mark is furious at his father for leaving him all these years to care for his mother. Mark states that he feels hopeless and he is frightened at the prospect of the family meeting.

Dr. Chandler wonders how the mother must be feeling. If Mark leaves for college, she'll lose her main support. She's made a home for Mark all these years and must be tired of having to beg her ex-husband for money. The father could understandably be wondering if the mother isn't actually able to work and is taking advantage of him financially. Mark's father may be worried that his son has bipolar illness like his mother.

The next morning, Dr. Chandler orients the family to the session, thanking the parents for coming and acknowledging how awkward and difficult it is for a divorced people to come together with their former spouse at a family meeting. He underscores the importance of Mark's having the support and involvement of both of his parents. Dr. Chandler asks each family member what he or she thinks is going to happen in today's meeting and then offers his own expectations for the meeting. Dr. Chandler explains, "I'd like to hear from each family member about what you think are the major problems facing your family, and I will give you feedback, a summary, of what I think you're saying, to make sure that I understand. I want you to tell me if I've got it right or not." He adds, "We probably will not be solving major problems in today's meeting, but rather we can gain a clearer understanding of the family problems from everyone's perspective and, I hope, identify how best to address these problems." Each family member voices agreement with the process and goals.

Mark's mother starts the session, saying, "I'm very upset and so is Mark because Mark's father has abruptly decided to stop paying child support." She continues, "He didn't speak with me directly but rather told Mark to tell me about this change. I've always tried to be fair. I've never gone to a lawyer. We've always worked it out." As the mother lists her complaints about Mark's father, Dr. Chandler realizes that he has made a mistake, allowing the mother to have the floor first. He is aware of the father's growing discomfort and hostility. As the mother explains her concerns, Dr. Chandler waits for an appropriate opening and checks in with the father. Dr. Chandler says to the father, "I know that it's very difficult to sit and listen to these complaints, but you'll have a chance to share your concerns in just a minute." It is important that Dr. Chandler offer brief reassurance to help the criticized family member tolerate the discussion. The growing tension in the room is somewhat dissipated. The father sits quietly while the mother finishes articulating her concerns.

When Dr. Chandler asks the father about his concerns, the father states, "I'm very angry. I've just been given a list of charges that I have to answer. I don't think I want to have any part of this." Dr. Chandler stays calm and again acknowledges, "I know it is difficult for you to listen to the concerns of your ex-wife, but it is important, if things are going to improve for Mark, that the two of you talk about these problems together as Mark's parents." Dr. Chandler encourages the father to share his concerns. Dr. Chandler's empathetic acknowledgment of how difficult it is to discuss these issues helps the father participate in the family meeting. After a long pause, the father says, "I have many concerns, the most important being Mark's illness and hospitalization. I'm worried about Mark's future, that his depression may be the start of an illness like his mother's." At this point, Dr. Chandler makes a point of underscoring that the parents are in agreement on the issues affecting Mark's health and are, in the meeting today, working together.

The father continues, "She also uses Mark as a go-between and does not talk with me directly." The parents then begin to argue about how much time the father should be spending with Mark. Dr. Chandler allows this disagreement to continue for a short while and does not overreact to the escalating tension resulting from the parents' sparring. Dr. Chandler understands that it is hard for these divorced parents to be together in this forum and is ready to intervene if the arguing begins to interfere with the progress of the session. After a few minutes, the parents become aware of having taken over the meeting with their argument and, with mixed feelings of guilt, frustration, and lingering anger, stop their charges and countercharges.

Dr. Chandler asks Mark about his concerns, and Mark states tearfully, "I can't take you guys constantly bickering and putting me in the middle. I've tried to ask you to stop but you go on and on. You both act stupid." Mark's parents listen attentively as Mark cries and tells them how distressed he is. Dr. Chandler asks Mark how long this has been going on. Mark, encouraged by Dr. Chandler's interest, answers, "They've been fighting and putting me in the middle for 12 years, since I was just a little kid, and I'm sick of it. I can't take it anymore." Dr. Chandler gives Mark feedback, "Mark, for the past 12 years you've been caught between your parents, who argue and put you in the middle of their arguments, is that right?" Mark loudly answers "Yes!" Mark's parents are both sullen and look downward. Dr. Chandler asks them, "What do you think about what Mark has said?" Both parents quietly respond that they didn't know that Mark was so troubled by their arguing. Dr. Chandler adds, "And being put in the middle of your arguments."

Dr. Chandler addresses Mark: "You said that your parents act stupid. How do your mother and father act stupid?" Mark replies, "My mother gets all hysterical and starts crying for me to talk to my father about whatever is going on, and my Dad gets mad, says he doesn't want to hear it, and just walks away and won't talk to me." Dr. Chandler asks Mark," Have you tried to tell your parents about this?" Mark responds, "Many times. They just don't listen." Dr. Chandler focuses on the parents. "It's very distressing for children when divorced parents fail to communicate directly with each other and use their children to communicate to their ex-spouse. Many times, divorced spouses have unresolved issues; and unfortunately, these issues can get in the way of their working together and can become barriers between parent and child. It's very difficult for everyone, especially the children." By the forlorn look on both of the parents' faces, Dr. Chandler realizes that Mark's words are finally being heard by his parents. Dr. Chandler knows that at this point Mark's words are more powerful than anything he might say to the parents, so he lets them sink in.

After a few minutes, Dr. Chandler asks Mark if he has other concerns. Mark is able to tell his father, "I miss seeing you, Dad." Mark's father agrees. "I've missed seeing you as well. I've been on sabbatical and out of the country, but I'm around more now, so we can see each other." Mark responds, "Are we going to be able to go away this summer?" Mark's father replies, "Yes, let's plan to go to the beach house for a couple of weeks." For the first time in the meeting, Mark smiles.

Dr. Chandler asks if there are other family concerns to address in today's meeting. Mark's mother addresses his father, "I'd like to talk about your saying you are going to stop child support." Mark's father responds sarcastically, "I think you can begin to make some financial contribution." Mark's mother snaps back, "Why did you tell Mark you weren't going to pay child support?" Mark's father explains, "I asked Mark to tell you that I couldn't pay last month's child support on time, not that I won't continue to pay. I've been late with only last month's payment." Mark's mother seems surprised.

Dr. Chandler asks, "Is this true, Mark's father has been late with only last month's child support payment?" Both Mark and his mother say that it is true. Dr. Chandler uses the opportunity to point out that clear and direct communication between the parents could have saved everyone a great deal of distress. Mark's father says again, "I think she needs to get a job and begin making a financial contribution." Mark's mother responds, "I'm not in a position to get a job at this time." As the meeting comes to a close, Dr. Chandler wisely says to Mark's parents, "On the issue of Mark's mother's getting a job, at this point you see things very differently, so I suggest that for now you agree to disagree on this issue. Our time for today's meeting is running out, and I want to review the discharge plan for Mark."

The family and Dr. Chandler review the discharge plan for Mark, and Dr. Chandler asks the parents what they are taking away from the meeting. Both mother and father say that they will communicate directly with each other from now on and that they are sorry for the pain they have caused Mark. Mark says that he feels the meeting was helpful, but then asks his father if he is mad at him. Mark's father reassures Mark that he is not angry at him. The father says he is glad he came to the meeting.

Lessons Learned

The goals for the meeting have been met: Mark's father came to the meeting and the parents agreed to communicate directly with each other rather than putting Mark in the middle. Raising the consciousness of the family members helped them take an important step toward more open communication and problem solving. This is best illustrated by Mark's poignant telling of his story in his own words. This case example is another illustration of the power for change that is released when family members come together and are given the opportunity to discuss their problems in an atmosphere of dignity and mutual respect. Such a meeting provides the support needed for a family to take the first steps toward resolving problems. There were no fancy, sophisticated family therapy techniques in this family meeting. Dr. Chandler realized the power of being able to convene a family meeting and allowing a forum for family members to discuss their problems with a neutral facilitator.

Dr. Chandler's diplomatic efforts enabled both parents to attend the meeting. While he was unable to meet with each parent individually before meeting with them together, he was fair and equitable in dealing with the parents and quickly compensated for not allowing the father to speak first. He successfully created a neutral environment by his vigilance and frequent sensitive interventions. He repeatedly reminded the family that it is important to truly listen to each other and try to find common ground when possible. He also supported Mark by pointing out that when parents communicate through their child, it places a great burden on the child.

Dr. Chandler also played an important role as educator by explaining how divorce restructures the family unit and how ongoing conflicts between divorced parents affect the children. Divorced parents need to be reminded that, while they are no longer husband and wife, they are forever bound together as parents through the existence of their child (Prosky 1991) and that the single best predictor of children's adjustment after divorce is the quality of the ex-spouses' co-parental relationship (Goldsmith 1982). While the majority of divorced parents are deeply concerned about their children's adjustment following the divorce, many have little understanding of how their postdivorce behavior affects their children.

What if the session had not gone well and had been fraught with arguing and defensiveness? Before ending the meeting, Dr. Chandler would have attempted to educate the parents about how their arguing and putting Mark in the middle were hurting Mark and contributing to his problems. If the meeting had ended with the parents still at war, Dr. Chandler would have used the events of the family meeting to help Mark understand the fallibility of his parents and begin to separate himself from their ongoing conflicts.

SUMMARY

The resident who understands the anxieties and fears of family members is more empathetic and effective in family meetings. Family skills supervision guides the resident in understanding the perspective of each family member. This is the groundwork needed for the resident to form an alliance with the family and to develop a treatment plan that involves the family. The supervisor also guides the resident in setting realistic goals for the family meeting. When the resident has an understanding of the fears and anxieties of each family member and can structure the family meeting accordingly, the meeting is more likely to be successful.

PART FIVE

The Larger System

CHAPTER TEN

Risk Management
and the Family

PATRICIA R. RECUPERO, J.D., M.D.

This chapter discusses some risk-management practices for psychiatrists working with inpatients and their families. By conscientiously respecting all parties' legal rights and adhering to the standard of care, psychiatrists help avoid adverse outcomes for patients and litigation against themselves and their institution. While it is impossible to eliminate all legal risks from the practice of psychiatry, working with families affects the types and degrees of risk involved and may present opportunities for reducing risk. Particular areas of concern include informed consent, confidentiality of patients and their family members, alienation of family members, suicidal or dangerous patients, and prescription medicines. The American Psychiatric Association encourages involving family members in evaluation and psychoeducation in both inpatient and outpatient settings, with the patient's permission (APA 2006). This discussion outlines important lessons using relevant case law and gives practical suggestions for decreasing risk in psychiatric inpatient care.

WHY RISK MANAGEMENT?

Like all other doctors, while striving for the best therapeutic outcome for their patients, psychiatrists must fulfill legal obligations to protect patients' and families' privacy and safety, as well as honoring ethical and professional duties. Involving families in patient care is important for risk management. The psychiatrist's failure to recognize the important role families play in the assessment and treatment of a patient is often the root cause of malpractice lawsuits lodged against a psychiatrist. Numerous lawsuits have documented psychiatrists' failures to listen to family members, and often it is the excluded or disgruntled family member who initiates the litigation. As several forensic psychiatrists have noted, "Bad feelings combined with a bad outcome often lead to litigation" (Gutheil, cited in Simon 1992, p. 292). Therefore, involving families in the treatment process minimizes the risk of adverse outcomes by reducing the likelihood of the "bad feelings" that could provoke a lawsuit.

Good patient care and risk-management measures are enhanced by the involvement of family members at three stages of care: (1) the initial assessment, (2) the planning of treatment, and (3) the planning of discharge. During the initial assessment, the psychiatrist gathers information from family members about the patient's history and previous treatment outcomes. During treatment planning, family members should collaborate with the treatment team in developing a plan that is acceptable to all parties. Finally, during discharge planning, psychiatrists should ensure that family members are actively engaged in providing a safe, supportive environment for the patient. In the case of short inpatient stays, there is usually the opportunity for only one family meeting, and consultation on these three phases occurs in the single family meeting. This chapter describes three specific risk situations—suicidal patients, dangerous patients, and prescription medications—and gives practical suggestions to decrease risk in each case. First, general comments about informed consent and confidentiality are reviewed.

INFORMED CONSENT

Informed consent is a valuable tool for risk management. In the orientation at the beginning of the family meeting, the physician discusses the goals for the meeting and clarifies the expectations of each family member. Documenting these elements as well as the family's agreement to proceed by recording them in the doctor's notes on the meeting enhances the risk-management potential of the meeting. The crucial feature of a valid informed consent, for the purpose of risk management, is the aspect of dialogue and understanding among all present (Schuck 1994). During this discussion, the physician should explain that the purpose of the meeting is to obtain a history, answer questions from the family, and discuss the treatment plan.

If the family enters family therapy, a new informed consent process is appropriate. Family therapy carries unique risks and benefits of which families may not be aware (Jensen, Josephson, and Frey 1989). As with any treatment, psychiatrists should obtain their patients' informed consent before the treatment (Noah 2002).

PATIENT'S CONFIDENTIALITY

Confidentiality is the sine qua non of psychiatric treatment. The duty to protect a patient's confidentiality may pose a challenge when a psychiatrist is conducting a meeting with the patient's family. Even when a patient consents to a family meeting, the psychiatrist should take care not to unnecessarily reveal the patient's confidential information. In the case of *Eckhardt v. Charter Hospital of Albuquerque* (1997), the director of a counseling center learned that a patient undergoing treatment at the center had been physically abused by her alcoholic husband. The director then mentioned to the patient's husband that she knew him to be an "abusive alcoholic." The patient, put at greater physical risk by this breach of confidence, subsequently succeeded in a lawsuit against the counseling center director, alleging wrongful disclosure of confidential information. This case illustrates the general rule that psychiatrists should never disclose information learned from patients unless compelled by law to do so. There are other cases in which psychiatrists have been held liable for unauthorized disclosure of confidential information to a patient's spouse (e.g., *MacDonald v. Clinger* 1982); there are even cases of disclosure to other psychiatrists (*Berry v. Moench* 1958) who later revealed the information to family members.

Psychiatrists must walk a fine line between disclosing a patient's secrets and working with the family. Adolescents in particular create difficult treatment dilemmas. While many therapists would disclose information about risky behaviors, such as drug use or promiscuity, to an adolescent's parents, such disclosures undermine adolescent autonomy and may have a chilling effect on a patient's willingness to be open and honest with the psychiatrist

(Marrus 1998). In many cases, parents already know or suspect their children's risky behaviors, and family meetings can provide a safe, therapeutic forum in which young people can confess such problems to their parents with the support of the neutral psychiatrist. The psychiatrist can facilitate the revelation and discussion by asking general questions and normalizing typical adolescent behaviors, saying, for example, "Adolescents often join with peer groups and may engage in risky behaviors. Do you have any concerns about your son's being involved with peers whom you don't approve of?" The parents and adolescent are then free to discuss their concerns without having to be responsible for initiating the discussion.

FAMILY MEMBERS' CONFIDENTIALITY

A psychiatrist can be held liable for wrongful disclosure of privileged information and for breach of confidential relations if he or she divulges information about a family member learned during a family meeting. In the case of *Mrozinski v. Pogue* (1992), the court rejected the psychiatrist's assertion that he had no duty to protect the family member's confidentiality, explaining their reasoning as follows: "The strongest public policy considerations militate against allowing a psychiatrist to encourage a person to participate in joint therapy, to obtain his trust and extract all his confidences and place him in the most vulnerable position, and then abandon him on the trash heap of lost privilege" (*Mrozinski*, at 408). Thus, the physician must consider what information about family members to divulge as well as to whom.

However, there are circumstances in which the disclosure of confidential information is appropriate (e.g., threats of bodily harm to specific individuals and suspected child or elder abuse). Residents must learn how to handle the disclosure of child abuse or elder abuse in family meetings. Family members who are empathetically engaged by the resident may "report themselves," that is, call the appropriate protective agency and request help. Families thus engaged by the physician are far less likely to sue for a false report. At the beginning of the family meeting, the resident can discuss the legal obligation to report known or suspected child or other abuse and the necessity to notify the appropriate state agency. If abuse is disclosed, the resident can then facilitate that report either during or immediately after the meeting. Although some scholars have argued that warnings of the practitioner's legal obligation may have a chilling effect, inhibiting patients' candor and honesty (Marrus 1998), a failure to warn patients and families about mandated reporting may more dramatically undermine trust in the psychiatrist-patient relationship, resulting in "bad feelings" that the patient or family has been betrayed or deceived.

ALIENATING FAMILY MEMBERS

Psychiatrists often hear negative information from patients about their families, such as allegations of physical or sexual abuse. Psychiatrists should be careful not to react to hearsay information and should strive to remain neutral. The treating physician should ask him- or herself, "Do I know the full story? Have I listened to the family members? What have I learned from them about my patient?" Under some circumstances, family members have claimed injury by the therapist when the patient has not. In the 1990s, courts and newspapers were replete with accounts of "false memory syndrome" lawsuits brought by family members against therapists who allegedly had helped their patients to recover repressed memories of childhood abuse. These false-memory suits involved widely ranging claims, including malpractice, negligence, defamation, intentional infliction of emotional distress, breach of contract, and invasion of privacy (Lipton 1999). In some of these cases, patients recant, deciding that the "recovered" memories were not real memories at all, but fabrications. Furthermore, even when patients have not recanted, family members harmed through "recovered memories" have been successful in suing the therapist for consequences, including loss of job, divorce, and alienation from family members (*Ramona v. Ramona* 1994; *Ramona v. Superior Court of Los Angeles County* 1997). Family members may also bring loss of consortium claims for interference with spousal relationships or malpractice claims for intentional interference with parent-child relationships (Kisch 1996).

Therefore, when recording notes, it is prudent to avoid recording the names of third parties and to avoid making potentially libelous statements. "Explored patient's memories of abuse" is more appropriate than "patient reported having sex with his father on July 4, 1965"; "patient reports stressful relationship with mother" is less risky than "patient's mother is sociopathic and abusive." Even if amicable relationships cannot be restored, family members can develop an empathetic understanding of the patient's suffering while disputing certain of the patient's beliefs. Meeting with the family may help establish some common ground that will allow both parties to work together. In some cases, the family and patient may have to "agree to disagree" about the past and focus on future treatment goals.

SPECIFIC RISKS
Suicidal Patients

The completed suicide of a patient is one of the most common claims in psychiatric malpractice suits (Melonas, cited in Bender 2003, p. 11; Williams 1997). These claims are usually brought by the next of kin (Bender 2003). The "special relationship" between a psychiatrist and a patient gives rise to a special duty to use due care to prevent the patient from committing suicide (Kussman 2004). Due care, according to current practice standards, usually requires family involvement (APA 2003, p. 35). While psychiatrists do not owe a duty of care to family members as part of the doctor-patient relationship, involving them may reduce the likelihood that surviving family members of completed suicides will sue under state wrongful death statutes (Simon 1992).

Ignoring family members is among the surest ways to create the "bad feelings" that provoke a lawsuit. For example, a woman who had urged her brother to seek psychiatric treatment initiated a lawsuit against his mental health treatment providers (*O'Sullivan v. Presbyterian Hospital* 1995). Although she had telephoned the treatment team numerous times, no member of the team requested any information from her about her brother's history. As a result, the treatment team failed to diagnose an episode of major depressive disorder and instead treated the patient for anxiety. The patient subsequently committed suicide. A court-appointed expert wrote, "information from the patient's personal physician, *from his family*, and perhaps from others might have been helpful in assuring that an accurate portrayal of the patient and his background were going into the diagnostic formulation" (emphasis added). Family members can provide information that a depressed, withdrawn, or suspicious patient is unable to provide, and families of potentially suicidal patients may have information that could prove helpful in diagnosis and treatment.

It is prudent to conduct a risk assessment of the household when discharging a patient. A doctor who released a violent, suicidal patient to the custody of his mother was held liable to the patient's mother and daughter for failing to inquire into the security of the patient and the availability of weapons at the mother's house, where the patient later shot and killed himself (*Martin v. Smith* 1993). *The risk of suicide among recently discharged psychiatric inpatients is at least 200 times greater than that for the general population* (Davidson 1999). An important part of discharge planning is to assess the safety of the environment to which the patient is going and to ask about the availability of weapons and the security of all medicines. There is often a need to balance the patient's confidentiality with safety concerns. For example, one patient confided to the resident that she had a stash of medications at home that her husband did not know about which she was keeping "just in case." At the family meeting, the next day, the patient was given ample opportunity to bring up this issue. She failed to do so. When the patient asked the attending physician about discharge, he stated that there was a safety issue at home that needed to be cleared up. The husband immediately asked the patient what the treatment team's concerns were and reluctantly the patient divulged the location of the stash of pills. In this case, protecting the patient outweighed confidentiality duties.

A risk-reduction strategy that offers multiple benefits is to provide, during a family meeting before discharge, psychoeducation about the warning signs of recurring suicidal ideation. The understanding and cooperation of family members in patient care after discharge helps protect against the significant risk of suicide. It is important to explain to family members the role they have in the care of the patient after discharge. Keeping follow-up appointments and understanding what to do if their loved one shows signs of noncompliance are key components of this role. Family members should understand their responsibilities and should indicate their agreement to the patient's release from the hospital. Documentation of the family's understanding, informed consent, and compliance with appropriate safety measures is essential.

Dangerous Patients

The Tarasoff case (*Tarasoff v. Regents of the University of California* 1976) legally recognized the psychiatrist's duty to protect known potential victims of violent or dangerous patients. The news media are peppered with stories of individuals murdering or attacking family members, and psychiatric records—whether they be charts, session notes, or taped communications—often become the focus of scrutiny (*Menendez v. Superior Court of Los Angeles County* 1992).

One case highlights the importance of risk management during the initial assessment of a violent patient. A daughter of a woman murdered by her common-law husband brought a wrongful death suit alleging that psychiatrists failed to obtain a dangerous patient's past medical record and failed to warn the woman, who was a probable victim (*Jablonski v. United States* 1983). Although the victim had expressed fears to two psychiatrists before the murder, they neglected to request the patient's past medical record, which would have indicated a diagnosis of "schizophrenic reaction, undifferentiated type, chronic, moderate; manifested by homicidal behavior toward his wife" (*Jablonski* at 393–94) and that he had on numerous occasions tried to kill her. Lacking this information and ignoring a warning from police officers, the psychiatrists found no basis to hospitalize the patient involuntarily. They also neglected to adequately warn the victim, as their warnings to her were "unspecific and inadequate under the circumstances" (*Jablonski* at 398).

When assessing, treating, or discharging violent patients, the psychiatrist can take two crucial steps to reduce risk: (1) investigate the basis of family members' fears and concerns, and (2) provide specific, practical warnings to probable victims (e.g., "Your life may be in danger. If you'd like to get a restraining order, here is the phone number to call. Here is a phone number for a domestic violence hotline, and here are some phone numbers and locations for local battered women's shelters"). In some circumstances, assistance with these referrals may be necessary.

Prescription Medications

Many malpractice lawsuits against psychiatrists involve allegations about "bad outcomes" from medications (Cash 2004). During the assessment phase, the psychiatrist may learn valuable information from family members about a patient's or family's history of substance abuse or adverse reactions to certain medications. In *Argus v. Sheppegrell* (1985), a doctor prescribed amphetamines and barbiturates to a young woman who was pursuing a modeling career. The patient's mother advised the doctor that her daughter was addicted to the prescriptions. Ignoring the mother's information, the doctor continued to prescribe addictive substances for the young woman, who subsequently died from a lethal overdose, giving rise to the parents' lawsuit against the physician. Had the doctor taken the mother's concerns seriously, the young woman's fatal overdose might have been prevented. Patients with a dual diagnosis carry an increased risk, as they are more likely to be suicidal, violent, and dangerous to third parties (e.g., as drunk drivers) (Recupero 2000). These increased risks should prompt the physician to have a family meeting to discuss risks, warning signs, and actions for family members to take if their loved one shows signs of relapse or impairment.

The family also plays an important role in the management of medications after discharge. Current practice suggests that in cases of alcohol dependence, family members supervise the administration of Antabuse and help with dietary guidelines to avoid use of alcohol in cooking. For depression, if a patient is taking a monoamine oxidase inhibitor (MAOI), families must learn MAOI dietary restrictions and potentially lethal drug interactions. While good practice may suggest that only a week's supply be dispensed, economic realities, such as co-pays, may move the psychiatrist to write prescriptions for larger amounts. Families can be helpful by taking custody of the large number of pills and releasing them on a daily or weekly basis. Such a family strategy reduces the likelihood of a patient's hoarding medication for a suicide attempt.

SUMMARY

Knowledge of legal concerns educates the resident about important aspects of treatment. For example, listening to a patient's family members and recognizing them as valuable sources of information about the patient is an important and easy way to reduce risk in psychiatric practice. Families can provide information that increases the likelihood of an accurate diagnosis or early detection of harmful behaviors such as substance abuse and self-injurious behavior. Family members usually want to be helpful; they appreciate guidance that may lessen the likelihood of harm to their loved ones. The resident needs the patient's written consent to talk to the family about the patient but does not need permission to *listen* to the family. Listening to the family, taking their fears and concerns seriously, teaching them how to help keep their loved one safe, being careful with therapies that may alienate them, monitoring countertransference reactions, respecting ethical boundaries, and respecting confidentiality are important aspects of patient care. The resident should document the needs and concerns expressed by the family and the steps taken to ensure the safety of not only the patient but others as well. Courts may interpret a failure to completely document treatment information as evidence that a psychiatrist fell below an acceptable standard of care (Rychik and Lowenkopf 2000). Good documentation and good rapport with family members perform a protective function against adverse incidents and increase both the efficacy and the enjoyment of inpatient psychiatric practice. When the resident is able to work well with patients' families, there is a greater likelihood of a good outcome for all.

CHAPTER ELEVEN

Family-Based Services after Hospitalization

This chapter summarizes the desires and needs of families and describes family-based services in the community. The provision of family-oriented care will require changes in the organization of services in hospitals and mental health centers and in the training of staff, especially psychiatrists.

WHAT FAMILIES WANT

When families are asked what they want from the mental health care system, they state that they want not lengthy and intensive interventions but family care that focuses on building rapport and communication (Rose, Mallinson, and Walton-Moss 2004). Families in a study of this subject identified several problems with treatment: poor-quality care, conflict with health professionals about treatment, and lack of a role for families in the treatment of their relatives. In addition, African American families identified isolation of their communities from the mental health system. Adolescents emphasized that they also serve as or would like to be involved as caregivers and identified their needs for support.

Family members state that they benefit from help that focuses on specific problems, such as how to manage disruptive patient behavior, which allows them to develop an increased sense of control. This leads to a reduction in family arguments, fewer missed days at work or school, and less disruption of the household (Reinhard 1994). The National Alliance for the Mentally Ill (NAMI) conducted a survey of families and consumers of psychiatric services and found that the level of family satisfaction was related to the amount of information the family received from health care providers. The survey results showed that 72 percent of family members received some information about their relative's illness (Marshall and Solomon 2000). However, most of these family members were not involved in any discussion of the treatment plan. NAMI recommended improved collaboration among health care provider and consumer and family.

WHAT FAMILIES NEED

In studies of family caregivers of inpatients with chronic mental illness, 70 percent reported depressive symptoms as well as impaired social, family, physical, and emotional functioning (Heru and Ryan 2002; Heru, Ryan, and Vlastos 2004). Less than 30 percent of these caregivers received help from other relatives, and only 5 percent had sought help from organizations such as NAMI. These difficulties are collectively referred to as *caregiver burden*, which describes the way in which a caregiver's life-style has been altered by the role of caregiver. *Objective burden* describes the effects of caregiving on the health, finances, and activities of the caregiver; *subjective burden* is the extent to which a relative feels burdened, and it includes worrying, tension, insomnia, and resentment. Caregivers who understand that their relative's behavior is caused by illness and not by willfulness report the least burden (Wendel et al. 2000). Psychoeducational interventions that improve the caregiver's knowledge of the illness reduce subjective burden (Dixon et al. 2001; Reinares et al. 2004). The caregiver's quality of life also improves with services that support, educate, and involve family members (Corring 2002). When caregivers receive emotional support from family and friends, especially when they know that other families struggle with similar problems, they develop a stronger sense of family competence (Johnson 2000). Thus, the provision of services to the family members of inpatients can significantly reduce caregiver burden and enhance coping skills.

The needs of the children of parents with a psychiatric illness have been neglected by adult psychiatry. Psychiatrists and psychologists tend to be interested in these children only if they show psychiatric or psychological symptoms but not as the offspring or caregivers of ill parents or siblings. Aldridge and Becker (2003) present the perspectives of these children, their parents, and professionals with whom they have worked, based on in-depth research with 40 families. Resources have been created by some children and teenagers who themselves understand young caregivers' need for information and the health profession's need for information about them. They have published a book (Gowen 2001) and they run a website (www.youngcarers.com), which is maintained by the Children's Society in the United Kingdom. In the United States, the Family Studies Team of the South Central Mental Illness Research, Education and Clinical Center (MIRECC), in Oklahoma City, has recently produced guides for teenagers with a parent who has PTSD (Sherman and Sherman 2006a) or chronic mental illness (Sherman and Sherman 2006b).

Young people report that they are ignored by professionals and that they want to understand what is happening to their parent or sibling and to be part of the decisions made about their family. They report that they want to be respected, included, and acknowledged. The needs of young children range from a child who is coping well and is hungry for information to a child whose own health is threatened by the situation and who needs support, treatment, and perhaps protection (Falkov and Lindsey 2002). The extent of a child's vulnerability depends on many factors, including the specific diagnoses of the parent, whether the illness is occurring at a critical developmental stage for the child, the amount of social stigmatization caused by the illness, and the degree of geographical or cultural isolation.

It is important that clinicians who work with adult patients ask about the experiences of children in the home. Ascertaining this information from the children themselves may take some extra effort. Often children are excluded from family meetings because they are in school when the meetings are held or because parents want to "protect" the children. Clinicians can explain to the parents that their children may have questions that are important to them, that they may have unfounded fears that are distressing them and distorting their understanding of the circumstances, and that they may benefit from education and support. When children visit their parent in hospital, age-appropriate literature and contact information can be made available to them. This area of family work is now gathering international recognition.

When health professionals were asked their concerns about the mental health system's efficacy at meeting the needs of families, they identified system-based barriers, professional practice–based barriers, and family-based barriers to the provision of good health care (Rose, Mallinson, and Walton-Moss 2004). It is of significance that they also reported a lack of training and resources to deal with complex family issues. The scarcity of such professional help has led family members to develop their own services.

FAMILY-DEVELOPED SERVICES

Family members of patients have developed sophisticated self-help groups through the National Alliance for the Mentally Ill. The most widely used family education model is the Family-to-Family Education Program (FFEP), formerly the Journey of Hope Education Program, which was developed in the early 1990s. This twelve-week program is run by family members who are specifically trained as group leaders, using a structured, scripted manual (Burland 1998). The program is free and is supported by a combination of grassroots donations and state mental health funds. Caregivers receive information about mental illnesses, treatments and medication, and rehabilitation. They learn self-care and communication skills as well as problem-solving and advocacy strategies, and they develop insight into their own response to mental illness (NAMI-MD 1998). FFEP classes are held in the community and are open to anyone with a family member who has serious and persistent mental illness, whether or not the ill person is receiving treatment. Currently, FFEP is offered in 45 U.S. states, Puerto Rico, two Canadian provinces (British Columbia and Ontario), and three regions in Mexico. It has more than 3,000 volunteer teachers and 250 trainers of new teachers, and it plans to continue international expansion.

A few studies have been done on the successfulness of these programs. In one, family members who attended this program felt less displeasure and worry about their ill family member and felt more empowered in the community, in their family, and with the service system than before the program (Dixon et al. 2004). This study found significant benefit from attending the program when comparing family members on the waitlist (three months before entering FFEP), at baseline (at the beginning of FFEP), immediately after FFEP, and six months after FFEP was completed. Another study showed that family members who participate in family education programs have greater knowledge and self-efficacy and are more satisfied with the patient's treatment than those who do not participate (Solomon et al. 1997). It has also been shown that overall patient and family satisfaction is increased when families are involved in the assessment and treatment of patients (Doherty 1995).

WHAT CAN HOSPITALS AND MENTAL HEALTH CENTERS DO?

Hospitals and community mental health services need to develop the fiscal structure and support to administer psychoeducational programs for family members. One excellent program that can be adapted to any clinical situation was developed by the Oklahoma City Veterans Affairs (VA) Medical Center (Sherman 2003). This program, called the Support and Family Education (SAFE) Program: Mental Health Facts for Families, consists of a 14-session family psychoeducational curriculum. Each 90-minute workshop occurs once a month, and participants attend whenever they wish. The program has six major goals: to teach caregivers about the symptoms and course of mental illnesses; to afford family members the opportunity to ask questions about psychiatric disorders and treatment options; to reduce the stigma of mental illness by providing a forum in which to discuss concerns and obtain support from peers; to publicize the availability of mental health services at the medical center; to help family members understand the importance of early intervention for their loved one and of open, timely communication with providers; and to link family members with support programs both at the medical center and through community resources, including the local branch of NAMI. The VA has distributed 130 copies of SAFE manuals to VA networks across the country, facilitating the adoption of the program. In addition, the University of Oklahoma Information Technology Group created a website (http://www.ouhsc.edu/safeprogram) that contains the entire manual. The site includes detailed outlines of the 14 sessions, specific publicity strategies for attracting family attendance, and a literature review attesting to the positive impact of educating families.

In the community, the viability of establishing family psychoeducational group treatment was studied in 15 mental health agencies in Maine and 51 in Illinois (McFarlane et al. 2001). Nearly all the Maine sites implemented such services, whereas only a few of the Illinois sites did. Several possible reasons have been suggested for this, including the fact that the Maine's trainees expressed less skepticism about family psychoeducation and more interest in receiving supervision and consultation. In Maine there was also widespread local support before and during implementation of the programs and more federal funding made available for support than in Illinois. Thus, successful implementation is enhanced by consensus building and adequate funding.

Hospitals can work with residency programs to provide improved training for psychiatric residents. The new impetus from the ACGME regarding core competencies may provide an added incentive to develop family-oriented care. The challenges that trainees face in learning to work with families should be seen as part of the normal development of the resident and should be specifically addressed during the training of residents (Heru and Drury 2006). The expectation that all mental health professionals will learn how to work with families should be made explicit throughout the hospital environment. An institutional commitment from the residency director and department chair that families should be included in patient care can set the tone for trainees. Supervisors do not need to be family psychiatrists, but they need to be able to apply a family-oriented approach to patient care.

SUMMARY

When the resident understands the perspective of the family and what they face in the community, he or she will be more empathetic and helpful to individual families and can help support family-based organizations. The resident should educate patients and families and refer them to community resources. With an increased awareness of the needs of patients and families, the resident is in a better position to become a patient and family advocate, in the hospital and in the community at the local, state, and even national levels.

GAP Checklist for Evaluating Competency in Family-Interview Skills

Interview of a Family

(Please rate on scale of 1–5, with 3 as expected level of performance.)

The resident is able to:	poor				excellent
Identify the role of family in presenting problem	1	2	3	4	5
Identify the family's developmental stage/transition	1	2	3	4	5
Identify any pertinent cultural/special situations	1	2	3	4	5
Identify the family's strengths and resources	1	2	3	4	5
Be supportive, respectful, and collaborative	1	2	3	4	5
Show balanced concern for each person's point of view	1	2	3	4	5
Understand family interactions	1	2	3	4	5
Manage expression of affect	1	2	3	4	5
Assess the family using the GARF scale	1	2	3	4	5
Provide psychoeducation	1	2	3	4	5
Intervene in basic problems	1	2	3	4	5
Know when to refer complicated problems	1	2	3	4	5

Interview of a Couple

The resident:

Joined with both members	Yes	No
Reviewed the structure and purpose of the evaluation	Yes	No
Obtained information from referring doctor	Yes	No
Obtained information about:		
the current living arrangements of the couple	Yes	No
names and ages of children	Yes	No
others living in the household	Yes	No
Asked about ethnicity/culture	Yes	No
Asked for each partner's version of the presenting problem	Yes	No
Obtained a couples history	Yes	No
Obtained an individual history from each	Yes	No
Obtained a three- or four-generation genogram	Yes	No
Identified issues in the time line of the couple that may be central to the problem (e.g., job stress, birth of children, illness or death of significant people)	Yes	No
Inquired about substance abuse	Yes	No

Did the resident:

Use language that was appropriate to both partners?	Yes	No
Ask at least one question about family strengths?	Yes	No
Allow or request an enactment?	Yes	No
Control the session appropriately (encourage both to speak, end arguments when appropriate)?	Yes	No
Maintain connection to both partners?	Yes	No
Demonstrate empathy and active listening?	Yes	No

Source: Adapted from Group for the Advancement of Psychiatry, Committee on the Family, 2006.

References

Accreditation Council for General Medical Education (ACGME). 2004. www .acgme.org.

Aldridge, J., and Becker, S. 2003. *Children Caring for Parents with Mental Illness: Perspectives of Young Carers, Parents and Professionals.* Bristol, U.K.: Policy Press. (Available in U.S. via International Specialized Book Services, 920 N.E. 58th Avenue, Suite 300, Portland, Oreg. 97213; 503-287-3093, 1-800-944-6190.)

American Psychiatric Association (APA). 2000. *Diagnostic and Statistical Manual of Mental Disorders,* fourth edition, text revision. Washington, D.C.: American Psychiatric Association.

American Psychiatric Association (APA). 2003. Practice guidelines for the assessment and treatment of patients with suicidal behaviors. *American Journal of Psychiatry* Suppl. 160 (November):35.

American Psychiatric Association (APA). 2006. Practice guidelines for the psychiatric evaluation of adults, 2nd ed. *American Journal of Psychiatry* 163, 6 Suppl. (June):6–7.

American Psychiatric Association (APA), Work Group on Bipolar Disorder. 2002. Practice guidelines for the treatment of patients with bipolar disorder, revision. *American Journal of Psychiatry* 159, 4 Suppl.

American Psychiatric Association (APA), Work Group on Depression. 2000. Practice guidelines for the treatment of patients with depression, supplement. *American Journal of Psychiatry* 157, 4 Suppl.

American Psychiatric Association (APA), Work Group on Schizophrenia. 2004. Practice guidelines for the treatment of patients with schizophrenia, second edition. *American Journal of Psychiatry* 161, 2 Suppl.

Anderson, C.M., Hogarty, G.E., and Reiss, D.J. 1980. Family treatment of adult schizophrenic patients: A psychoeducational approach. *Schizophrenia Bulletin* 65:490–505.

Antonovsky, A. 1987. *Unraveling the Mystery of Health.* San Francisco: Jossey-Bass.

Argus v. Sheppegrell, 472 So.2d 573 (La. 1985).

Asen, E. 2002. Outcome research in family therapy. *Advances in Psychiatric Treatment* 8:230–38.

Barrett, P., Healy-Farrell, L., and March, J.S. 2004. Cognitive-behavioral family treatment of childhood obsessive-compulsive disorder: A controlled trial. *Journal of the American Academy of Child and Adolescent Psychiatry* 43 (1):46–62.

Barrett, P., Rasmussen, P., and Healy, L. 2001. The effects of childhood obsessive-compulsive disorder on sibling relationships in late childhood and early adolescence: Preliminary findings. *Australian Journal of Educational and Developmental Psychology* 17:82–102.

Barrett, P., Shortt, A., and Healy, L. 2002. Do parent and child behaviors differentiate families whose children have obsessive-compulsive disorder from other clinic and non-clinic children? *Journal of Child Psychology and Psychiatry* 43:597–607.

Barrowclough, C., and Hooley, J. 2003. Attributions and expressed emotion: A review. *Clinical Psychological Review* 23:849–80.

Barrowclough, C., Johnston, M., and Tarrier, N. 1994. Attributions, expressed emotion, and patient relapse: An attributional model of relatives' response to schizophrenic illness. *Behavior Therapy* 25:67–88.

Bateson, G.B., Jackson, D., Haley, J.J., and Weakland, J. 1956. Towards the theory of schizophrenia. *Behavioral Science* 1:251–64.

Beavers, W.R., and Hampson, R.B. 1990. *Successful Families: Assessment and Intervention.* New York: W.W. Norton.

Bender, E. 2003. Psychiatrists can minimize malpractice suit anxiety. *Psychiatric News* 38 (August):11.

Berkman, L.F., Leo-Summers, L., and Horwitz, R. 1992. Emotional support and survival after myocardial infarction: A prospective, population-based study of the elderly. *Annals of Internal Medicine* 117:1003–9.

Berman, E., and Heru, A.M. 2005. Family systems training in psychiatric residencies. *Family Process* 44:321–35.

Berry v. Moench, 331 P.2d 814 (Utah 1958).

Bertalanffy, L.V. 1968. *General System Theory: Foundations, Development, Applications.* New York: Braziller.

Bertrando, P., Beltz, J., Bressi, C., Clerici, M., Farma, T., Invernizzi, G., and Cazzullo, C.L. 1992. Expressed emotion and schizophrenia in Italy: A study of an urban population. *British Journal of Psychiatry* 161:223–29.

Bhugra, D., and McKenzie, K. 2003. Expressed emotion across cultures. *Advances in Psychiatric Treatment* 9:342–48.

Bowen, M. 1978. *Family Therapy in Clinical Practice.* New York: Jason Aronson.

Brendel, D. 2005. Healing Psychiatry: The need for pragmatism. American Psychiatric Association Symposium 20D, Atlanta.

Brewin, C.R., MacCarthy, B., Duda, K., and Vaughn, C.E. 1991. Attribution and expressed emotion in the relatives of patients with schizophrenia. *Journal of Abnormal Psychology* 100:546–54.

Brown, G.W., Carstairs, G.M., and Topping, G. 1958. Post-hospital adjustment of chronic mental patients. *Lancet* 2:685–89.

Brown, G.W., and Rutter, M. 1966. The measurement of family activities and relationships: A methodological study. *Human Relations* 19:241–63.

Budman, S.H., and Gurman, A.S. 1988. *Theory and Practice of Brief Therapy*. New York: Guilford Press.

Burland, J. 1998. Family-to-family education course. Arlington, Va.: National Alliance for the Mentally Ill.

Butzlaff, R.L., and Hooley, J.M. 1998. Expressed emotion and psychiatric relapse. *Archives of General Psychiatry* 55:547–52.

Calabrese, J.R., Hirschfeld, R.M., Frye, M.A., and Reed, M.L. 2004. Impact of depressive symptoms compared with manic symptoms in bipolar disorder: Results of a U.S. community-based sample. *Journal of Clinical Psychiatry* 65 (11):1499–504.

Campbell, T.L. 2003. The effectiveness of family interventions for physical disorders. *Journal of Marital and Family Therapy* 29 (2):263–81.

Canive, J.M., Sanz-Fuentenebro, J., Vasquez, C., et al. 1996. Family psychoeducational support groups in Spain: Parents distress and burden at nine-month follow-up. *Annals of Clinical Psychiatry* 8 (2):71–79.

Cash, C. 2004. A few simple steps can avert medical errors. *Psychiatric News* 39 (February):10.

Caspi, A., McClay, J., Moffitt, T.E., Mill, J., Martin, J., Craig, I.W., Taylor, A., and Poulton, R. 2002. Role of genotype in the cycle of violence in maltreated children. *Science* 297 (5582):851–54.

Clarkin, J.F., Carpenter, D., Hull, J., Wilner, P., and Glick, I. 1998. Effects of psychoeducational intervention for married patients with bipolar disorder and their spouses. *Psychiatric Services* 49:531–33.

Cohen, A.N., Hammen, C., Henry, R.M., and Daley, S.E. 2004. Effects of stress and social support on recurrence in bipolar disorder. *Journal of Affective Disorders* 82 (1):143–47.

Corring, D. 2002. Quality of life: Perspectives of people with mental illnesses and family members. *Psychiatric Rehabilitation Journal* 25 (4):350–59.

Coyne, J.C., Rohrbaugh, M.J., Shoham, V., Sonnega, J.S., Nicklas, J.M., and Cranford, J.A. 2001. Prognostic importance of marital quality for survival of congestive heart failure. *American Journal of Cardiology* 88:526–29.

Dare, C., Eisler, I., Russell, G., et al. 2001. Psychological therapies for adults with anorexia nervosa: A randomized controlled trial of outpatient treatments. *British Journal of Psychiatry* 178:216–22.

Davidson, L. 1999. Discharge decision making with recently suicidal inpatients. *Directions in Psychiatry* 19:339–46.

DeMaria, R., Weeks, G., and Hof, L. 1999. *Focused Genograms*. Philadelphia: Brunner/Mazel.

Dixon, L., Luckstead, A., Stewart, B., Burland, J., Brown, C.H., Postrado, L., McGuire, C., and Hoffman, M. 2004. Outcomes of the peer-taught 12-week family-to-family education program for severe mental illness. *Acta Psychiatrica Scandinavica* 109 (3):207–15.

Dixon, L., Stewart, B., Burland, J., Delahanty, J., Licksted, A., and Hoffman, M. 2001. Pilot study of the effectiveness of the family-to-family education program. *Psychiatric Services* 52 (7):965–67.

Dodge, K.A., and Pettit, G.S. 2003. A biopsychosocial model of the development of chronic conduct problems in adolescence. *Developmental Psychology* 39 (2):349–71.

Doherty, W.J. 1995. Boundaries between patient and family education and family therapy. *Family Relations* 44:353–58.

Dyche, L., and Zayas, L.H. 1995. The value of curiosity and naivete for the cross-cultural psychotherapist. *Family Process* 34:389–99.

Eckhardt v. Charter Hospital of Albuquerque, 953 P.2d 722 (N.M. Ct. App. 1997).

Engel, G.L. 1977. The need for a new medical model: A challenge for biomedicine. *Science* 196:129–36.

Engel, G.L. 1978. The biopsychosocial model and the education of health professionals. *Annals of the New York Academy of Sciences* 310:169–87.

Epstein, N.B., and Bishop, D.S. 1981. Problem-centered systems therapy of the family. In A.S. Gurman and D.P. Kniskern, eds., *The Handbook of Family Therapy*. Bristol, Pa.: Brunner/Mazel, pp. 444–82.

Epstein, N.B., Ryan, C.E., Bishop, D.S., et al. 2003. The McMaster Model: View of healthy family functioning. In F. Walsh, ed., *Normal Family Processes*, third edition. New York: Guilford, pp. 138–60.

Falkov, A., and Lindsey, C. 2002. Patients as parents: Addressing the needs including the safety of children whose parents have mental illness. Council Report CR 105. London Royal College of Psychiatrists.

Foley, D.L., Eaves, L.J., Wormley, B., Silberg, J.L., Maes, H.H., Kuhn, J., and Riley, B. 2004. Childhood adversity, monoamine oxidase a genotype, and risk for conduct disorder. *Archives of General Psychiatry* 61 (7):738–44.

Fromm-Reichman, F. 1948. Notes on the development of treatment of schizophrenics by psychoanalytic psychotherapy. *Psychiatry* 11:263–73.

Fudge, E., Falkov, A., Kowalenko, N., and Robinson, P. 2004. Parenting is a mental health issue. *Australasian Psychiatry* 12 (2):166.

Gabbard, G., and Kay, J. 2001. The fate of integrated treatment: Whatever happened to the biopsychosocial psychiatrist? *American Journal of Psychiatry* 158 (12): 1956–63.

Garmezy, N. 1991. Resiliency and vulnerability to adverse developmental outcomes associated with poverty. *American Behavioral Scientist* 34:416–30.

Geist, R., Heinmaa, M., Stephens, D., Davis, R., and Katzman, D.K. 2000. Comparison of family therapy and family group psychoeducation in adolescents with anorexia nervosa. *Canadian Journal of Psychiatry* 45 (2):173–78.

Ghaemi, S.N. 2003. *The Concepts of Psychiatry: A Pluralistic Approach to the Mind and Mental Illness.* Baltimore: Johns Hopkins University Press.

Gitlin, M., Swendsen, J.T., Heller, T., and Hammen, C. 1995. Relapse and impairment in bipolar disorder. *American Journal of Psychiatry* 152:1635–40.

Glick, I.D., Clarkin, J.F., Haas, G.L., and Spencer, J.H., Jr. 1993. Clinical significance of inpatient family intervention: Conclusions from a clinical trial. *Hospital and Community Psychiatry* 44 (9):869–73.

Goldsmith, J. 1982. The post-divorce family system. In F. Walsh, ed., *Normal Family Processes.* New York: Guilford, pp. 297–330.

Gowen, S., ed. 2001. *Visible Voices: Young People's Ideas Annual.* London: Community Links.

Group for the Advancement of Psychiatry (GAP), Committee on the Family. 1996. Global Assessment of Relational Functioning (GARF): Background and rationale. *Family Process* 35:155–72.

Group for the Advancement of Psychiatry (GAP), Committee on the Family. 2006. Family skills for general psychiatry residents: Meeting ACGME core competency requirements. *Academic Psychiatry* 30 (1):69–78.

Grunes, M.S., Neziroglu, F., and McKay, D. 2001. Family involvement in the behavioral treatment of obsessive-compulsive disorder: A preliminary investigation. *Behavior Therapy* 32:803–20.

Guarnaccia, P.J., and Parra, P. 1996. Ethnicity, social status and families' experiences of caring for a mentally ill family member. *Community Mental Health Journal* 32:243–60.

Gunderson, J.G., Berkowitz, C., and Ruiz-Sancho, A. 1997. Families of borderline patients: A psychoeducational approach. *Bulletin of the Menninger Clinic* 61 (4):446–57.

Gunderson, J.G., and Lyoo, I. 1997. Family problems and relationships for adults with borderline personality disorder. *Harvard Review of Psychiatry* 4:272–78.

Guttman, H.A., Feldman, R.B., Engelsmann, F., Spector, L., and Buonvino, M. 1999. The relationship between psychiatrists' couple and family therapy training experience and their subsequent practice profile. *Journal of Marital and Family Therapy* 25 (1):31–41.

Hayhurst, H., Cooper, Z., Paykel, E.S., Vearnals, S., and Ramana, R. 1997. Expressed emotion and depression: A longitudinal study. *British Journal of Psychiatry* 171:439–43.

Heacock, C. 2004. Psychiatrists versus psychopharmacologists. *Psychiatric Times,* August, p. 13.

Heru, A.M. 2000. Family functioning, burden and reward in the caregiving for chronic mental illness. *Families, Systems and Health* 18 (1):91–103.

Heru, A.M., and Drury, L. 2006. Overcoming barriers in working with families. *Academic Psychiatry* 30(5):379–84.

Heru, A.M., and Ryan, C.E. 2002. Depressive symptoms and family functioning in the caregivers of recently hospitalized patients with chronic/recurrent mood disorders. *International Journal of Psychosocial Rehabilitation* 7:53–60.

Heru, A.M., Ryan, C.E., and Vlastos, K. 2004. Quality of life and family functioning in caregivers of patients with mood disorders. *Psychiatric Rehabilitation Journal* 28 (1):67–71.

Hibbs, E.D., Hamburger, S.D., Lenane, M., Rapoport, J.L., Kruesi, M.J., Keysor, C.S., and Goldstein, M.J. 1991. Determinants of expressed emotion in families of disturbed and normal children. *Journal of Child Psychology and Psychiatry* 32 (5):757–70.

Hinrichsen, G.A., Adelstein, L., and McMeniman, M. 2004. Expressed emotion in family members of depressed older adults. *Aging and Mental Health* 8 (4):355–63.

Hollon, S.D., and Fawcett, J. 1995. Combined medication and psychotherapy. In G.O. Gabbard ed., *Treatments of Psychiatric Disorders*, second edition, vol. 1. Washington, D.C.: American Psychiatric Press, pp. 1221–36.

Hooley, J.M., and Campbell, C. 2002. Control and controllability: Beliefs and behavior in high and low expressed emotion relatives. *Psychological Medicine* 32 (6):1091–99.

Hooley, J.M., and Hoffman, P.D. 1999. Expressed emotion and clinical outcome in borderline personalities. *American Journal of Psychiatry* 156 (10):1557–62.

Hooley, J.M., Orley, J., and Teasdale, J.D. 1986. Levels of expressed emotion and relapse in depressed patients. *British Journal of Psychiatry* 148:642–47.

Hooley, J.M., and Teasdale, J.D. 1989. Predictors of relapse in unipolar depressives: Expressed emotion, marital distress and perceived criticism. *Journal of Abnormal Psychology* 3:229–35.

Ivanovië, M., Vuletië, Z., and Bebbington, P. 1994. Expressed emotion in the families of patients with schizophrenia and its influence on the course of illness. *Social Psychiatry and Psychiatric Epidemiology* 29:61–65.

Jablonski v. United States, 712 F.2d 391 (9th Cir. 1983).

Jackson, D.D. 1957. A note on the importance of trauma in the genesis of schizophrenia. *Psychiatry* 20:181–84.

Jenkins, J.H., and Karno, M. 1992. The meaning of expressed emotion: Theoretical issues raised by cross-cultural research. *American Journal of Psychiatry* 149 (1):9–21.

Jenkins, J.H., and Schumacher, J.G. 1999. Family burden of schizophrenia and depressive illness: Specifying the effects of ethnicity, gender and social ecology. *British Journal of Psychiatry* 174:31–38.

Jensen, P.S., Josephson, A.M., and Frey, J., III. 1989. Informed consent as a framework for treatment: Ethical and therapeutic considerations. *American Journal of Psychotherapy* 43 (July):378–86.

Johnson, E.D. 2000. Differences among families coping with serious mental illness: A qualitative analysis. *American Journal of Orthopsychiatry* 70 (1):126–34.

Johnson, J.G., Cohen, P., Kasen, S., Smailes, E., and Brook, J.S. 2001. Association of maladaptive parental behavior with psychiatric disorder among parents and their offspring. *Archives of General Psychiatry* 58:453–60.

Johnson, S., and Kizer, A. 2002. Bipolar and unipolar depression: A comparison of clinical phenomenology and psychosocial predictors. In I. Gotlib and C. Hammen, eds., *Handbook of Depression*. New York: Guilford Press, pp. 141–65.

Johnson, S., Winett, C., Meyer, B., Greenhouse, W., and Miller, I. 1999. Social support and the course of bipolar disorder. *Journal of Abnormal Psychology* 108:558–66.

Kamal, A. 1995. Variables in expressed emotion associated with relapse: A comparison between depressed and schizophrenic samples in an Egyptian community. *Current Psychiatry* 2:211–16.

Karlson, E.W., Liang, M.H., Eaton, H., Huang, J., Fitzgerald, L., Rogers, M.P., and Daltroy, L.H. 2004. A randomized clinical trial of a psychoeducational intervention to improve outcomes in systemic lupus erythematosus. *Arthritis and Rheumatism* 50 (6):1832–41.

Karno, M., Jenkins, J.H., de la Selva, A., Santana, F., Telles, C., Lopez, S., and Mintz, J. 1987. Expressed emotion and schizophrenic outcome among Mexican-American families. *Journal of Nervous and Mental Disease* 175:143–51.

Kasanin, J., Knight, E., and Sage, P. 1934. The parent-child relationship in schizophrenia. *Journal of Nervous and Mental Disease* 79:249–63.

Kavanaugh, D.J. 1992. Recent developments in expressed emotion and schizophrenia. *British Journal of Psychiatry* 160:601–20.

Keitner, G.I., Archambault, R., and Ryan, C.E. 2003. Family therapy and chronic depression. *Journal of Clinical Psychology / In Session* 59:873–84.

Keitner, G.I., Drury, L.M., Ryan, C.E., Miller, I.W., Norman, W.H., and Solomon, D.A. 2002. Multifamily group treatment for major depressive disorder. In W.R. McFarlane, ed., *Multifamily Group Treatment for Severe Psychiatric Disorders*. New York: Guilford, pp. 244–67.

Keitner, G.I., and Miller, I.W. 1990. Family functioning and major depression: An overview. *American Journal of Psychiatry* 147:1128–37.

Keitner, G.I., Ryan, C.E., Miller, I.W., Kohn, R., Bishop, D.S., and Epstein, N.B. 1995. Role of the family in recovery and major depression. *American Journal of Psychiatry* 152 (7):1002–8.

Keitner, G.I., Ryan, C.E., Miller, I.W., and Norman, W.H. 1992. Recovery and major depression: Factors associated with twelve-month outcome. *American Journal of Psychiatry* 149 (1):93–99.

Keitner, G.I., Ryan, C.E., Solomon, D.A., Kelley, J.E., and Miller, I.W. 2003. Family therapy and family functioning in patients with mood disorders. American Psychiatric Association Annual Meeting. May, San Francisco.

Keller, M.B., McCullough, J.P., Klein, D.N., Arnow, B., Dunner, D.L., Gelenberg, A.J., Markowitz, J.C., Nemeroff, C.B., Russell, J.M., Thase, M.E., Trivedi, M.H., and Zajecka, J. 2000. A comparison of nefazodone, the cognitive behavioral-analysis system of psychotherapy, and their combination for the treatment of chronic depression. *New England Journal of Medicine* 342:1462–70.

Kimand, E.Y., and Miklowitz, D.J. 2004. Expressed emotion as a predictor of outcome among bipolar patients undergoing family therapy. *Journal of Affective Disorders* 82 (3):343–52.

King, S., and Dixon, M.J. 1999. Expressed emotion and relapse in young schizophrenia outpatients. *Schizophrenia Bulletin* 25:377–86.

Kisch, W.J. 1996. From the couch to the bench: How should the legal system respond to recovered memories of childhood sexual abuse? *American University Journal of Gender and the Law* 5 (Fall):207–46.

Klass, P. 1987. *A Not Entirely Benign Procedure: Four Years as a Medical Student.* New York: Signet.

Kleinman, A. 1988. *Patients and Healers in the Context of Culture.* Berkeley: University of California Press.

Kopelowicz, A., Zarate, R., Gonzalez, V., López, S.R., Ortega, P., Obregon, N., and Mintz, J. 2002. Evaluation of expressed emotion in schizophrenia: A comparison of Caucasians and Mexican Americans. *Schizophrenia Research* 55:179–86.

Krysan, M., Moore, K.A., and Zill, N. 1990. *Identifying Successful Families: An Overview of Constructs and Selected Measures.* Washington, D.C.: Child Trends Inc. and U.S. Department of Health and Human Services, Office of the Assistant Secretary for Planning and Evaluation.

Kussman, P.C. 2004. Liability of doctor, psychiatrist, or psychologist for failure to take steps to prevent patient's suicide. 81 *American Law Reports* 5th, 167.

Laffel, L.M., Vangsness, L., Connell, A., Goebel-Fabbri, A., Butler, D., and Anderson, B.J. 2003. Impact of ambulatory, family-focused teamwork intervention on glycemic control in youth with type 1 diabetes. *Journal of Pediatrics* 142 (4): 409–16.

Lee, S., Colditz, G.A., Berkman, L.F., and Kawachi, I. 2003. Caregiving and risk of coronary heart disease in U.S. women: A prospective study. *American Journal of Preventive Medicine* 24 (2):113–19.

Leff, J., and Vaughn, C. 1985. *Expressed Emotion in Families.* New York: Guilford Press.

Leff, J., Vearnals, S., Wolff, G., Alexander, B., Chisholm, D., Everitt, B., Asen, E., Jones, E., Brewin, C.R., and Dayson, D. 2000. The London Depression Intervention Trial. Randomized controlled trial of antidepressants v. couple therapy in the treatment and maintenance of people with depression living with a partner: Clinical outcome and costs. *British Journal of Psychiatry* 177:95–100.

Leff, J., Wig, N.N., Ghosh, A., Bedi, H., Menon, D.K., and Kuipers, L. 1987. Influence of relatives' expressed emotion on the course of schizophrenia in Chandigarh. *British Journal of Psychiatry* 151:166–73.

Lefley, H.P. 1992. Expressed emotion: Conceptual, clinical and social policy issues. *Hospital and Community Psychiatry* 43:591–98.

Lidz, T., Cornelison, A.R., Fleck, S., et al. 1957. The intrafamilial environment of the schizophrenic patient. Part 2: Marital schism and marital skew. *American Journal of Psychiatry* 114:241–48.

Linehan, M.M., Armstrong, H.E., Suarez, A., Allmon, D., and Heard, H.L. 1991. Cognitive-behavioral treatment of chronically parasuicidal borderline patients. *Archives of General Psychiatry* 48:1060–64.

Lipton, A. 1999. Recovered memories in the courts. In Sheila A. Taub, ed., *Recovered Memories of Child Sexual Abuse: Psychological, Social, and Legal Perspectives on a Contemporary Mental Health Controversy*. Springfield, Ill. Charles C. Thomas, pp. 165–210.

López, S.R., Hipke, K.L., Polo, A.J., Jenkins, J.H., Karno, M., Vaughn, C., and Snyder, K.S. 2004. Ethnicity, expressed emotion, attributions, and course of schizophrenia: Family warmth matters. *Journal of Abnormal Psychology* 113 (3):428–39.

Luborsky, L., Diguer, L., Luborsky, E., Singer, B., Dickter, D., and Schmidt, K.A. 1993. The efficacy of dynamic psychotherapies: Is it true that "everyone has won and all must have prizes"? In N.E. Miller, L. Luborsky, J.P. Barber, and J.P. Docherty, eds., *Psychodynamic Treatment Research: A Handbook for Clinical Practice*. New York: Basic Books, pp. 497–516.

Luthar, S., Cicchetti, D., and Becker, B. 2000. The construct of resilience: A critical evaluation and guidelines for future work. *Child Development* 71:543–62.

MacDonald v. Clinger, 84 A.D.2d 482 (N.Y.S. App. Div. 1982).

Magana, A., Goldstein, M., Karno, M., Miklowitz, D., Jenkins, J., and Falloon, R. 1986. A brief method for assessing expressed emotion in relatives of psychiatric patients. *Psychiatry Research* 17:203–12.

Marrus, E. 1998. Please keep my secret: Child abuse reporting statutes, confidentiality, and juvenile delinquency. *Georgetown Journal of Legal Ethics* 11 (Spring): 509–46.

Marsh, D.T., and Lefley, H.P. 1996. The family experience of mental illness: Evidence for resilience. *Psychiatric Rehabilitation Journal* 20 (2):3–12.

Marshall, T.B., and Solomon, P. 2000. Releasing information to families of persons with severe mental illness: A survey of NAMI members. *Psychiatric Services* 51 (8):1006–11.

Martin v. Smith, 438 S.E.2d 318 (W.Va. 1993).

McClain, T., O'Sullivan, P.S., and Clardy, J.A. 2004. Biopsychosocial formulation: Recognizing educational shortcomings. *Academic Psychiatry* 28:88–94.

McFarlane, W.R., and Deakins, S.M. 2002. Family-aided assertive community treatment. In W.R. McFarlane, ed., *Multifamily Groups in the Treatment of Severe Psychiatric Disorders*. New York: Guilford Press.

McFarlane, W.R., Dixon, L., Lukens, E., and Luckstead, A. 2003. Family psychoeducation and schizophrenia: A review of the literature. *Journal of Marital and Family Therapy* 29 (2):223–45.

McFarlane, W.R., McNary, S., Dixon, L., Hornby, H., and Cimett, E. 2001. Predictors of dissemination of family psychoeducation in community mental health centers in Maine and Illinois. *Psychiatric Services* 52 (7):935–42.

McGoldrick, M. 2005. Multicultural family conference presentation. Butler Hospital, Providence, R.I.

McHugh, P.R., and Slavney, P.R. 1998. *The Perspectives of Psychiatry*, second edition. Baltimore: Johns Hopkins University Press.

Menendez v. Superior Court of Los Angeles County, 834 P.2d 786 (Cal. 1992).

Miklowitz, D.J. 2004. The role of family systems in severe and recurrent psychiatric disorders: A developmental psychopathology view. *Development and Psychopathology* 16:667–88.

Miklowitz, D.J., George, E.L., Richards, J.A., and Suddath, R.L. 2003. A randomized study of family-focused psychoeducation and pharmacotherapy in the outpatient management of bipolar disorder. *Archives of General Psychiatry* 60:904–12.

Miklowitz, D.J., and Goldstein, M.J. 1997. *Bipolar Disorder: A Family-Focused Treatment Approach*. New York: Guilford Press.

Miklowitz, D., Goldstein, M., Nuechterlein, K., Snyder, K., and Mintz, J. 1988. Family factors and the course of bipolar affective disorder. *Archives of General Psychiatry* 45:225–31.

Miller, I.W., Kabacoff, R.I., Keitner, G.I., Epstein, N.B., and Bishop, D.S. 1986. Family functioning in the families of psychiatric patients. *Comprehensive Psychiatry* 27:302–12.

Miller, I.W., Keitner, G.I., Ryan, C.E., Solomon, D., Cardemil, E.V., and Beevers, C.G. 2005. Treatment matching in the posthospital care of depressed patients. *American Journal of Psychiatry* 162 (11):2131–38.

Miller, I.W., Keitner, G.I., Whisman, M.A., Ryan, C.E., Epstein, N.B., and Bishop, D.S. 1992. Depressed patients with dysfunctional families: Description and course of illness. *Journal of Abnormal Psychology* 101 (4):637–46.

Mohr, W.K., Lafuz, J.E., and Mohr, B. 2000. Opening caregiver minds: National Alliance for the Mentally Ill's (NAMI) provider education program. *Archives of Psychiatric Nursing* 14 (5):235–43.

Mottaghipour, Y., Pourmand, D., Maleki, H., and Davidian, L. 2001. Expressed emotion and the course of schizophrenia in Iran. *Social Psychiatry and Psychiatric Epidemiology* 36 (4):195–99.

Mrozinski v. Pogue, 423 S.E.2d 405 (Ga. App. 1992).

National Alliance for the Mentally Ill (NAMI)–MD. 1998. Family-to-family program. *NAMI-MD Connections* 1998 (from the 1997–98 annual report) (Summer):4.

National Family Caregivers Association. 1997. Booklet from Fortis Long Term Care, 501 Michigan St., Milwaukee, Wisc. 53203.

Noah, L. 2002. Informed consent and the elusive dichotomy between standard and experimental therapy. *American Journal of Law and Medicine* 28:361–408.

O'Connor, T.G., Deater-Deckard, K., Fulker, D., Rutter, M., and Plomin, R. 1998. Genotype environment correlations in late childhood and early adolescence: Antisocial behavioral problems and coercive parenting. *Developmental Psychology* 34 (5):970–81.

O'Farrell, T.J., and Fals-Stewart, W. 2000. Behavioral couples therapy for alcoholism and drug abuse. *Journal of Substance Abuse Treatment* 18:51–54.

O'Farrell, T.J., and Fals-Stewart, W. 2003. Alcohol abuse. *Journal of Marital and Family Therapy* 29 (1):121–46.

O'Farrell, T.J., Fals-Stewart, W., Murphy, M., and Murphy, C.M. 2003. Partner violence before and after individually based alcoholism treatment for male alcoholic patients. *Journal of Consulting and Clinical Psychology* 71 (1):92–102.

O'Farrell, T.J, Hooley J., Fals-Stewart, W., and Cutter, H.S.G. 1998. Expressed emotion and relapse in alcoholic patients. *Journal of Consulting and Clinical Psychology* 66 (5):744–52.

Okasha, A., el Akabawi, K., Snyder, W.A., Youssef, I., and el Dawla, A. 1994. Expressed emotion, perceived criticism, and relapse in depression: A replication in an Egyptian community. *American Journal of Psychiatry* 151:1001–5.

Olson, D.H. 1996. Clinical assessment and treatment interventions using the family circumplex model. In F.W. Kaslow, ed., *Handbook of Relational Diagnosis and Dysfunctional Family Patterns.* New York: Wiley, pp. 59–80.

O'Sullivan v. Presbyterian Hospital, 217 A.D.2d 98 (N.Y. App. Div. 1995).

Parker, G., and Hadzi-Pavlovic, D. 1990. Expressed emotion as a predictor of schizophrenic relapse: An analysis of aggregated data. *Psychological Medicine* 20:961–65.

Perlick, D., Clarkin, J.F., Sirey, J., Raue, P., Greenfield, S., Struening, E., and Rosenheck, R. 1999. Burden experienced by care-givers of persons with bipolar affective disorder. *British Journal of Psychiatry* 175:56–62.

Perlick, D.A., Rosenheck, R.A., Clarkin, J.F., Maciejewski, P.K., Sirey, J., Stuening, E., and Link, B.G. 2004. Impact of family burden and affective response on clinical outcome among patients with bipolar disorder. *Psychiatric Services* 55 (9): 1029–35.

Phillips, M., and Xiang, W. 1995. Expressed emotion in mainland China: Chinese families with schizophrenic patients. *International Journal of Mental Health* 25:54–75.

Priebe, S., Wildgrube, C., and Muller-Oerlinghausen, B. 1989. Lithium prophylaxis and expressed emotion. *British Journal of Psychiatry* 154:396–99.

Prosky, P. 1991. Expanding our vision of family after divorce. *Brown University Family Therapy Letter* 3 (5):1–6.

Pruchno, R., Patrick, J.H., and Burant, C.J. 1997. African-American and white mothers of adults with chronic disabilities: Caregiving burden and satisfaction. *Family Relations* 46:335–46.

Ramona v. Ramona, No. 61898 (Cal. Super. Ct. 1994).

Ramona v. Superior Court of Los Angeles County, No. B111565, 57 Cal. App. 4th 107 (Cal. Ct. App. 1997).

Rea, M.M., Tompson, M.C., Miklowitz, D.J., Goldstein, M.J., Hwang, S., and Mintz, J. 2003. Family focused treatment versus individual treatment for bipolar disorder: Results of a randomized clinical trial. *Journal of Consulting and Clinical Psychology* 71:482–92.

Recupero, P.R. 2000. Risk management and the dual-diagnosis patient. *Directions in Psychiatry* 20:287–99.

Reinares, M., Vieta, E., Colom, F., Martinez-Aran, A., Torrent, C., Comes, M., Goikolea, J.M., Benabarre, A., and Sanchez-Moreno, J. 2004. Impact of a psychoeducational family intervention on caregivers of stabilized bipolar patients. *Psychotherapy and Psychosomatics* 73 (5):312–19.

Reinhard, S.C. 1994. Living with mental illness: Effects of professional support and personal control on caregiver burden. *Research in Nursing and Health* 17 (2): 79–88.

Reiss, D., Cederblad, M., Pedersen, N.L., Lichtenstein, P., Elthammar, O., Neiderhiser, J.M., and Hansson, K. 2001. Genetic probes of three theories of maternal adjustment. Part 2: Genetic and environmental influences. *Family Process* 40 (3):261–72.

Reiss, D., Hetherington, E.M., Plomin, R., Howe, G.W., Simmens, S.J., Henderson, S.H., O'Connor, T.J., Bussell, D.A., Anderson, E.R., and Law, T. 1995. Genetic questions for environmental studies: Differential parenting and psychopathology in adolescence. *Archives of General Psychiatry* 52 (11):925–36.

Rolland, J. 1994. *Families, Illness, and Disability: An Integrative Treatment Model.* New York: Basic Books.

Rose, L.E., Mallinson, R.K., and Walton-Moss, B. 2004. Barriers to family care in psychiatric settings. *Journal of Nursing Scholarship* 36 (1):39–47.

Ross, L.E., Sellers, E.M., Gilbert-Evans, S.E., and Romach, M.K. 2004. Mood changes during pregnancy and the post-partum period: Development of a biopsychosocial model. *Acta Psychiatrica Scandinavica* 109:457–66.

Rotunda, R.J., West, L., and O'Farrell, T.J. 2004. Enabling behavior in a clinical sample of alcohol-dependent clients and their partners *Journal of Substance Abuse Treatment* 26 (4):269–76.

Rutter, M. 2005. How the environment affects mental health. *British Journal of Psychiatry* 186:4–6.

Ryan, C.E., Epstein, N.B., Keitner, G.I., Miller, I.W., and Bishop, D.S. 2005. *Evaluating and Treating Families: The McMaster Approach.* New York: Brunner/Routledge.

Rychik, A., and Lowenkopf, E.L. 2000. Reviewing medical malpractice and risk management issues. *Psychiatric Times* 7 (August). www.psychiatrictimes.com.

Sadler, J. 2005. Six Questions for Clinical Models. American Psychiatric Association Symposium 20E, Atlanta.

Scazufca, M., and Kuipers, E. 1996. Links between expressed emotion and burden of care in relatives of patients with schizophrenia. *British Journal of Psychiatry* 168:580–87.

Schuck, P.H. 1994. Rethinking informed consent. *Yale Law Journal* 103:899–959.

Sherman, M.D. 2003. Rehab rounds: The Support and Family Education (SAFE) Program: Mental health facts for families. *Psychiatric Services* 54 (1):35–37.

Sherman, M.D., and Sherman, D.M. 2006a. *Finding My Way: A Teen's Guide to Living with a Parent Who Has Experienced Trauma*. Woodbury, Minn.: Seeds of Hope Books.

Sherman, M.D., and Sherman, D.M. 2006b. *I'm Not Alone: A Teen's Guide to Living with a Parent Who Has Mental Illness*. Woodbury, Minn.: Seeds of Hope Books.

Simon, R. 1989. Family life cycle issues in the therapy system. In B. Carter and M. McGoldrick, eds., *The Changing Family Life Cycle: A Framework for Family Therapy*, second edition. Boston: Allyn & Bacon, pp. 108–18.

Simon, R.I. 1992. *Clinical Psychiatry and the Law*, second edition. Washington, D.C.: American Psychiatric Press.

Slovik, L.S., Griffith, J.L., Forsythe, L., and Polles, A. 1997. Redefining the role of family therapy psychiatric residency education. *Academic Psychiatry* 21:35–41.

Solomon, P., Draine, J., Mannion, E., et al. 1997. Effectiveness of two models of brief family education: Retention of gains by family members of adults with serious mental illness. *American Journal of Orthopsychiatry* 67:177–86.

Steketee, G., and Van Noppen, B. 2003. Family approaches to treatment for obsessive compulsive disorder. *Revista Brasileira de Psiquiatria* 25 (1):43–50.

Stinnet, N., and DeFrain, J. 1985. *Secrets of Strong Families*. Boston: Little Brown.

Stirling, J., Tantan, D., Thomas, P., Newby, D., Montague, L., Ring, N., and Rowe, S. 1993. Expressed emotion and schizophrenia: The ontogeny of E.E. during an 18-month follow-up. *Psychological Medicine* 23:771–78.

Tanaka, S., Mino, Y., and Inoue, S. 1995. Expressed emotion and the course of schizophrenia in Japan. *British Journal of Psychiatry* 167 (6):794–98.

Tarasoff v. Regents of the University of California, 551 P.2d 334 (Cal. 1976).

Telles, C., Karno, M., Mintz, J., et al. 1995. Immigrant families coping with schizophrenia: Behavioral family intervention v. case management with a low-income Spanish-speaking population. *British Journal of Psychiatry* 167 (4):473–79.

Thara, R. 2004. Twenty-year course of schizophrenia: The Madras Longitudinal Study. *Canadian Journal of Psychiatry* 49 (8):564–69.

Thase, M.E., Greenhouse, J.B., Frank, E., Reynolds, C.F., III, Pilkonis, P.A., Hurley, K., Grochocinski, V., and Kupfer, D.J. 1997. Treatment of major depression with psychotherapy or psychotherapy-pharmacotherapy combinations. *Archives of General Psychiatry* 54:1009–15.

Thornicroft, G., Colson, L., and Marks, I.M. 1991. An inpatient behavioral psychotherapy unit description and audit. *British Journal of Psychiatry* 158:362–67.

Tienari, P., Wynne, C., Sorri, A., Lahti, I., Läksy, K., Moring, J., Naarala, M., Nieminen, P., and Wahlberg, K.E. 2004. Long-term follow-up study of Finnish adoptees. *British Journal of Psychiatry* 184:216–22.

Valleni-Basile, L.A., Garrison, C.Z., Waller, J.L., Addy, C.L., McKeown, R.E., Jackson, K.L., and Cuffe, S.P. 1995. Incidence of obsessive-compulsive disorder in a community sample of young adolescents. *Journal of American Child and Adolescent Psychiatry* 35 (7):898–906.

van Furth, E.F., van Strien, D.C., Martina, L.M., van Son, M.J., Hendrickx, J.J., and van Engeland, H. 1996. Expressed emotion and the prediction of outcome in adolescent eating disorders. *International Journal of Eating Disorders* 20 (1):19–31.

Van Noppen, B., Steketee, G., McCorkle, B.H., and Pato, M. 1997. Group and multifamily behavioral treatment for obsessive compulsive disorder: A pilot study. *Journal of Anxiety Disorders* 11:431–46.

Vaughn, C.E., and Leff, J.P. 1976a. The measurement of expressed emotion in the families of psychiatric patients. *British Journal of Social and Clinical Psychology* 129:125–37.

Vaughn, C.E., and Leff, J.P. 1976b. The influence of family and social factors on the course of psychiatric illness: A comparison of schizophrenic and depressed neurotic patients. *British Journal of Psychiatry* 129:125–37.

Vaughn, C.E., Snyder, K.S., Jones, S., Freeman, W.B., and Fallon, I.R. 1984. Family factors in schizophrenic relapse: Replication in California of British research on expressed emotion. *Archives of General Psychiatry* 41:1169–77.

Vieta, E., and Colom, F. 2004. Psychological interventions in bipolar disorder: From wishful thinking to an evidence-based approach. *Acta Psychiatrica Scandinavica* Suppl. (422):34–38.

Wachtel, E., and Wachtel, P. 1986. *Family Dynamics in Individual Psychotherapy: A Guide to Clinical Strategies.* New York: Guilford.

Waterman, S. 2005. The Limitations of the Biopsychosocial Model. American Psychiatric Association Symposium 20A, Atlanta.

Wearden, A.J., Tarrier, N., Barrowclough, C., Zastowny, T.R., and Rahill, A.A. 2000. A review of expressed emotion research in health care. *Clinical Psychology Review* 20 (5):633–66.

Weber, T., McKeever, E., and McDaniel, S.H. 1985. A beginner's guide to the problem-oriented first family interview. *Family Process* 24:357–63.

Weerasekera, P. 1996. *Multiperspective Case Formulation: A Step towards Treatment Integration.* Malabar, Fla.: Kreiger Publishing.

Weihs, K., Fisher, L., and Baird, M. 2002. Families, health and behavior. *Families, Systems and Health* 20 (1):7–46.

Wendel, J.S., Miklowitz, D.J., Richards, J.A., and George, E.L. 2000. Expressed emotion and attributions in the relatives of bipolar patients: An analysis of problem-solving interactions. *Journal of Abnormal Psychology* 109 (4):792–96.

Werner, E.E. 1993. Risk, resilience, and recovery: Perspectives from the Kauai longitudinal study. *Development and Psychopathology* 5:503–15.

Williams, C.J. 1997. Fault and the suicide victim: When third parties assume suicide victim's duty of self-care. *Nebraska Law Review* 76:301–18.

Yalom, I.D. 1993. *Inpatient Group Psychotherapy.* New York: Basic Books.

Yan, L.J., Hammen, C., Cohen, A.M., Daley, S.E., and Henry, R.M. 2004. Expressed emotion versus relationship quality variables in the prediction of recurrence in bipolar patients. *Journal of Affective Disorders* 83 (2–3):199–206.

Yingling L., Miller, W.E., McDonald, A.L., and Galewater, S.T. 1998. *GARF Sourcebook: Using the Global Assessment of Relational Functioning.* Washington, D.C.: Brunner/Mazel, Taylor & Francis.

Zacher, P. 2005. The Biopsychosocial Model: Strengths versus Weaknesses Related to Assumptions about Good Scientific Categories. American Psychiatric Association Symposium 20B, Atlanta.

Index